THE DIABETES EXIT

How to Reverse Type 2 Diabetes

When Knowing What to Do Has Never Been Enough

Dwain Woode, MD

Endocrinologist • Woode Life Design™

Published by Woode Life Design™. Huntsville, Alabama. dwainwoode.com

First Edition. Printed in the United States of America.

A note on currency: The drug classes, clinical guidelines, and device models referenced in this book, including GLP-1 receptor agonists, reflect information current as of the publication date. This field is evolving rapidly. Readers should consult current prescribing information and their physician for the most up-to-date guidance.

ISBN (paperback): 979-8-9959156-0-7

For Blake.

The reason I do what I do.

For Charmaine.

Who never stopped believing.

ACKNOWLEDGMENTS

This book belongs to the patients first.

Over twenty years, thousands of people sat across from me in an exam room and trusted me with their fear, their confusion, and their most private numbers. Many of them told me stories they had never told anyone — about chocolate eggs and Sunday mornings and fathers who came home bearing candy bars. They did not know they were teaching me. I did not know yet that I needed to be taught. This book is what I learned from them, and it could not exist without their willingness to let me inside the real story of their lives. They are in every chapter, unnamed but unmistakable.

To my team at the Diabetes and Endocrine Wellness Center — you showed up every day inside a practice that was asking more of you than you knew, and you did it with excellence and care. Thank you for staying.

To the Accelerators — the community that gathered around this work before the work was finished — you were the proof of concept. You asked better questions than I expected, pushed back when the framework needed it, and reminded me every week why this matters. This book is partly yours.

To Charmaine.

You waited. Through the years I was hiding — from my patients, from my practice, from myself — you waited for me to show up. Not for the version of me who had it figured out. For me. You held the house and the family and the quiet belief that the man you married was still in there, still becoming, still worth waiting for. The exit I found was not only metabolic. The person who came back to you on the other side of it — present, awake, no longer under the raft — was only possible because you did not stop believing he existed. I owe you more than this page can hold. But I start here.

To Blake.

You gave me a reason I could not argue with. Every framework in this book, every early morning, every choice to keep going when it was easier not to — I made it because of what I want to be able to teach you. Not from a stage. Not from a book. From a life you can watch and a father who showed you, by the way he lived, what it means to be a man. What it means to face the thing you are afraid of. What it means to stop hiding and start building. You did not know you were doing this. You were just being my son. That was enough. That was everything.

The exit is real. I found it. These are the people who made it possible to come back and say so.

Dwain Woode, MD

Huntsville, Alabama

CONTENTS

PREFACE

Why I Finally Said It Out Loud

For most of my career, I was the doctor who treated diabetes. I was also the man who had it. For a long time, those two facts lived in completely separate rooms, and I made sure the door between them stayed shut.

I was diagnosed during medical school. Not after. During. In the middle of learning how the disease worked, while I was being trained to treat it in other people, I was carrying it myself. I went through residency knowing. I went through fellowship knowing. I opened my practice, sat across from thousands of patients, talked to them about their blood sugar and their medications and their future, and I said nothing. Not because I did not care about them. Because I was afraid of what they would think — a doctor who could not do the very thing he was asking them to do.

So I hid.

For years my wife Charmaine said something to me. Not in the way of an argument. Not dramatically. Just quietly, persistently, the way a person says a thing they believe when they know you are not ready to hear it. She would say: you need to talk about this. She was talking about my diabetes. About the weight, the numbers, the version of me who sat across from patients explaining what they should do while quietly doing the opposite at home. She saw what I could not bring myself to name. She waited for me to see it too. I do not think I fully understood, for a long time, what that waiting cost her, or what it meant that she kept believing the man she married would eventually show up.

I started a YouTube channel. General health content at first. Thyroid, wellness, the things a physician could talk about without revealing too much. I was comfortable in that lane. What I did not understand was that the content was about to start doing something to me that I had not planned on.

Because here is what happened. Alongside that content, I started making other kinds of videos. Creating a better version of yourself. Living from the center. The art of letting go. Identity, authenticity, what it means to build a life with intention. I sat at my desk week after week and taught those ideas to my audience. But I was also teaching them to myself. And something was changing. Every time I looked into that camera and said you have to stop hiding the thing that is holding you back, I was also talking to the man in the room.

I joined a video content coaching program. The goal was to figure out how to build something — how to find my lane, develop a message, show up consistently with a clear identity. I was trying all kinds of directions. General health. Wellness. Fine content. Content that did not quite fit.

A member of my coaching group asked me a question I was not ready for. He looked at what I was making and he said: you are an endocrinologist. That is unique. Why are you not planted there?

I did not have a good answer.

That question did not immediately change anything. What it did was create a space in me that I could not fill with what I had been making. The lane I had been in suddenly did not fit anymore.

Not long after that, separately, I had a conversation with a coach — a man who had been listening to my full story for the first time. The diagnosis. The years of hiding. The patients. The weight. The slow reversal. When I finished, he said: do you understand how powerful this story is? He did not mean the clinical framework. He meant the man. The endocrinologist who had been diabetic for decades and had not told anyone and had found his way out. He said people need to hear this.

I received it as a challenge I was not yet ready to accept. But I could not un-hear it.

The river took care of the rest.

One year, during my son's Spring Break, we went whitewater rafting. The rapids got rough. The raft tipped. I fell into the water and grabbed the perimeter rope — as instructed, as any reasonable person would. And the raft came over me. I was underneath it, holding on, unable to breathe. The thing I was clinging to for safety was the thing preventing me from getting air.

It wasn't until I had no air left — no options, no alternatives, no breath remaining — that I finally let go.

When I let go, I came to the surface.

Standing on the bank afterward, soaking wet and shaken, I understood something that I hadn't been able to articulate for most of my career: the thing I was holding onto was not keeping me safe. It was keeping me under. The denial. The shame. The silence. The habits I had built around all of it. I had been clinging to them the way I had clung to that rope — out of fear, long past the point where they were helping me.

I decided, standing there, that I was done being under the raft.

I started telling the story. In every space where I had not been able to say it before — my clinic, my community, my platform. The words I had not been willing to say in my own clinic for years finally came out: I am diabetic. I have had this disease for decades. I hid it. I found the exit. And I built the framework that made the reversal possible.

Every time I say it, something happens in the room. Not applause. Something quieter. Recognition. The person in the third row whose mother has been hiding the same thing. The man in the back who has not told his wife. The woman who has been managing her blood sugar alone for years and has been carrying, quietly, the belief that it is her fault.

I know what it feels like to sit in the chair on the other side of the desk. As a patient. As a man who hid. As someone who has been exactly where you are — holding on, going under, not yet able to let go.

The exit is real. I found it. But first I had to stop clinging to the thing that was keeping me under.

That is why I finally said it out loud.

That is why this book exists.

— D.W.

INTRODUCTION

The Exit Exists

I have been a doctor for most of my adult life. I have also been a man with type 2 diabetes for most of it. The first part you will see on the cover of this book. The second part I have only recently been able to say out loud. The Preface tells you the story of how I came to say it. Chapter One tells you the story of the teenager who taught me what it would cost to keep hiding it. This book exists in the space between those two stories — between the silence I lived inside for decades, and the framework I built once the silence finally broke.

My Grandmother Said No.

As a young child in Rose Hall Town, Guyana, I fell off the porch of our family home. The fall was bad enough that my family took me to the local doctor. He examined me and, in so many words, told my family to take me home and make me comfortable.

My grandmother, Rebecca, said no.

She sat by my bedside. She applied the remedies she knew. She prayed. She refused to accept the doctor's conclusion as the final word. And I recovered. Slowly, completely, against what the expert in the room had decided was possible.

I did not understand what she had done until I was around ten or eleven years old, when the story was told to me fully for the first time. That the doctor had given up. That she had not. That what happened to me was not just a recovery — it was a reminder that exits exist even when experts say they do not.

I have been looking for exits my entire life.

My mother left Guyana for the United States when I was one year old. She went ahead to build something better for our family. I stayed behind with my grandparents until I was seven, when I joined her in Brooklyn in the mid 1970s, a world as different from Rose Hall Town as any place could be.

On my first day of school at PS 256, my sister and I opened our mouths and our Guyanese accents came out. The teachers heard something unfamiliar and placed us in bilingual education — a program designed for children who did not speak English. We spoke English. It was our native language. But we found our way to the right room. We always did.

I first set out to be a pastor. Then a PhD candidate. I failed the qualifying exam. Multiple times. The depression arrived. I started teaching at a local college. On my third career, carrying the accumulated weight of not quite making it, I went to medical school determined that this would be the one that finally worked.

It almost did not. I dropped out. I came back. And then the board exams — the licensing exams required to practice medicine. I failed them. Not once. Three times. I passed on the fourth attempt.

All the while, food was there. Not because I was weak. Because I was human and exhausted and carrying more pressure than I had the tools to process. The weight climbed with every setback. And somewhere in those years — during my first year of medical school, — I went to my doctor because I was waking up at night to urinate, feeling constantly hungry, dragging through every day. He ran some tests. I went home and slept, not thinking much of it.

My wife woke me from sleep to tell me the doctor had called.

I had diabetes.

What changed everything was the day I finally let go.

Since my journey began, I lost 100 pounds. My A1C came down from above 14 to 5.8. I came off my diabetes medications. I started talking publicly — on my YouTube channel, in my practice, in my community — about the disease I had spent over two decades hiding. I built a framework for reversing diabetes that drew on everything I knew as a physician and everything I had lived as a patient. I walked my community through it the same way I had walked myself through it: one step at a time, no shame, no pretense.

And now I am writing this book.

Not because I have it all figured out. Not because the journey is finished. But because I know something now that I wish someone had told me twenty-five years ago, the morning my wife woke me from sleep with news that changed everything:

The exit exists.

If you are holding this book, you are probably sitting with something. Maybe you received a diagnosis recently and you are still in the shock of it. Maybe you have been living with this disease for years and you are not where you want to be and you are tired of not being where you want to be. Maybe you picked this up because someone you love is struggling and you do not know how to help them. Maybe you are a patient who has nodded at a doctor's instructions and gone home and done something different.

Whatever brought you here, I want you to hear this first, before anything else:

You are not failing at health. You have been carrying shame that was never yours to carry alone. The disease is real. The biology is real. The forces working against you every single day — the habits, the emotions, the environment, the food system designed to override your best intentions — are real. You are not weak. You are not a lost cause. You are not a bad patient.

You have just never been given the right design.

This book is that design. It is built on twenty-plus years of clinical practice, on the latest science of metabolic health and diabetes reversal, and on the lived experience of a physician who was hiding in the same room as his patients for over two decades — and who finally found his way out.

My grandmother sat by my bedside when the doctor had already moved on. She refused to accept that there was no exit.

I am doing the same thing now for you.

The exit exists. I found it. And I came back to show you the way out.

Let's begin.

Dwain Woode, MD

Huntsville, Alabama

HOW TO USE THIS BOOK

This book is organized in four parts.

Part One — Chapters One through Three — establishes the foundation. Why the exit exists. What has been happening in your body. And the four forces that have been driving your eating beneath the level of conscious choice. If you have ever known exactly what you should do and still not done it, Part One explains why.

Part Two — Chapters Four through Seven — is the clinical framework. The three pillars of diabetes reversal: decreasing insulin, suppressing appetite, and reducing sugar. And then the chapter that shows you how all three work together inside a real day in a real life.

Part Three — Chapters Eight through Ten — addresses the invisible forces. The emotional brain and its direct impact on blood sugar. The C.O.P.E. framework for the moments that have historically undone you. And the environment design that shapes your choices before the moment of choice arrives.

Part Four — Chapters Eleven and Twelve — is about what becomes possible. Chapter Eleven is about the people around you — the relational dimension of this work, and the language that has to change between you and the people who love you for any of the rest of it to land the way it should. Chapter Twelve covers the domains of life that open up when health is no longer the problem, and the architecture of a life that holds your health over the long term.

You can read this book straight through, beginning to end. That is how it was designed to be read.

You can also use it as a reference. If you are in the middle of a difficult moment and need the C.O.P.E. framework immediately, go to Chapter Nine. If you want to understand what your blood sugar is actually responding to, go to Chapter Eight. If you need to remember why the exit is real when it stops feeling real, go back to Chapter One.

The final section of this book contains quick reference guides for C.O.P.E. and the H.E.A.T. model, a recommended labs list to bring to your next appointment, and a full About the Author section. These are designed to be used — not just read once and forgotten.

One more thing before you begin.

If you are currently on medication for diabetes — particularly insulin or sulfonylureas — please work with your healthcare provider as you implement this framework. The goal of this book is to give you the framework, the language, and the tools to reverse type 2 diabetes — and to help you understand, for the first time, why everything you tried before was not enough. Most people who open this book are already on medication. Some are on one. Some are on several. Some are on insulin. That is not a failure state — that is exactly the starting point this framework is designed to work from, alongside whatever your healthcare provider has prescribed. That process needs to be managed carefully with your healthcare provider, because as your blood sugar improves, the medication doses that were calibrated for your previous metabolic state may become too high. That is a good problem to have. But it needs medical supervision.

A note on medication and remission: some medications — including certain newer diabetes drugs — are now prescribed not just to lower blood sugar but to protect the heart and kidneys. If you are on one of those medications for reasons beyond blood sugar control, your healthcare provider may recommend continuing it even after your glucose levels normalize. That does not mean you have not achieved reversal. Work with your healthcare provider to understand exactly what each medication is doing for you. The rest of what follows belongs entirely to you.

PART ONE

The Problem

CHAPTER ONE

The Lie You Were Told

"We can manage it."

I want to tell you about a patient I saw early in my practice. He was a teenager and he had diabetes. He and his parents had been coming to see me for a couple of years by that point, and we had been trying everything — adjusting his medications, talking through his diet, working with his family. His blood sugars were never where we needed them to be. Every appointment, we went through the same conversation. Every appointment, the numbers told the same story.

One afternoon they came in and I could see the frustration in the room before anyone said a word. The boy looked at the floor. His mother looked at me. I started going through the plan again — what we needed to try, what we needed to change, what he needed to do differently. And then he looked up and said something I was not expecting.

He said: y'all don't understand.

He was not being disrespectful. He was being honest. He was a teenager and he had been living with a disease that was much bigger than him, and the people around him kept telling him what to do, and nothing was working, and he was tired. And then he looked at me directly and asked: Doc, are you diabetic?

I said no.

I do not know exactly why I said it that way. I could tell you it was reflexive. I could tell you I was caught off guard. Both of those things were true. But the real answer is simpler and less comfortable: I was ashamed. I had been practicing medicine for years at that point, carrying a disease I had never spoken aloud, and I was afraid of what they would think — a doctor who could not do the very thing he was asking them to do.

So I said no. And we finished the appointment. And they left.

I went home and I could not let it go.

I called them and asked them to come back. When they sat down across from me again, I told them what had happened. I told them I had not been honest. I told them I had been living with diabetes since medical school, that I had been carrying it the whole time I was treating his, that I had not told anyone, and that I was sorry for lying to him in that room.

There was a long silence.

His mother said: you lied.

And then the boy looked at his mother and said something I have thought about nearly every day since.

He said: see, even the doctor's ashamed.

He was not accusing me. He was recognizing something. He was a teenager who had been told, in a hundred different ways, that his disease was a reflection of his character — that if he were stronger, more disciplined, more committed, he would not be sitting in an endocrinologist's office with blood sugars that would not cooperate. And here was the doctor sitting across from him, the one doing the telling, and even he had been hiding.

That is what shame does. It does not stay in the individual. It travels. It passes between the person sitting at the desk and the person sitting across from it. It lives in the silence between the question and the honest answer. It convinces people that the disease is the evidence of some failure of character, and then it ensures they carry it alone, because no one wants to display the evidence.

I have been thinking about that room for a long time. About what it would have meant if I had told him the truth the first time he asked. About how many of the patients I saw in the years before that conversation were carrying the same weight he was — not just the disease, but the belief that it was their fault, that they deserved to be ashamed of it.

And I have been thinking about what he gave me, without knowing he was giving me anything. He named the thing I had not been able to name. He was a teenager, and he understood something about this disease that most of the medical education I had received never addressed.

The shame is part of the disease. And until we name it, we cannot treat it.

There is something that happens in the moment you are told — something that does not change regardless of how it arrives.

It doesn't matter whether you were expecting it or whether it arrived without warning. It doesn't matter whether you heard it in a hospital room or in a routine follow-up appointment or — as I did — from your wife, who woke you from sleep to relay a message from your healthcare provider. The moment the word arrives, something shifts. Not just in your understanding of your health. In your understanding of your future.

You have diabetes.

Three words. And in three words, a story begins to write itself in your mind — a story built from everything you have ever heard about this disease. The relatives who lost limbs. The neighbor who went on dialysis. The images of insulin syringes and glucose monitors and a lifetime of vigilance against a body that has turned, in some fundamental way, against itself.

I remember sitting with that word and thinking, in the particular way that only a medical student with unfinished business and a fragile sense of his own future can think: my career is over. Not my health. My career. The shame and the diagnosis arrived together, tangled so tightly I couldn't separate them. I was supposed to be the doctor. Doctors don't get this. And if they do, they certainly don't tell anyone.

You may not have been a medical student when you were diagnosed. But I suspect you had your own version of that thought. Your own first story. Your own quiet reckoning with what this word meant for the life you had been building.

That story — the one that began the moment the word arrived — is what this chapter is about. Because I want to tell you something important: parts of that story are not true. And the parts that aren't true have been quietly shaping every decision you've made about your health ever since.

When I went back to my doctor after the diagnosis, he started me on metformin.

There wasn't much education. There wasn't a conversation about what had caused my blood sugar to rise, or what the trajectory of my condition might look like, or what I could do — beyond taking the medication — to change that trajectory. There was a prescription. There was a follow-up appointment. And there were four words I have heard from patients in my own exam room hundreds of times since:

"We can manage it."

Those words were not unkind. My doctor was not negligent. He was doing what physicians had been trained to do, saying what the medical consensus at the time supported, offering what the system he worked inside was designed to deliver. He was being honest with me about what he believed was possible.

But embedded in those four words was an assumption so large and so unexamined that neither of us noticed it: that management was the ceiling. That the goal was not to get better but to get stable. That diabetes, once arrived, had arrived permanently — and the best we could hope for was to keep it quiet.

I walked out of that office with a prescription and a future that felt like it had already been written. A future organized around monitoring and medication and the slow, careful management of a condition I would carry for the rest of my life.

What I did not walk out with — what almost no patient walks out with, even today — was the knowledge that there was another possibility entirely.

Nobody told me about the exit.

I want to tell you what happens next.

Not just for me. For almost everyone who gets that diagnosis and that prescription and walks out into a parking lot with a future that has just been quietly rearranged.

You do what you are told. You fill the prescription. You show up to the follow-up. You check your blood sugar with the frequency that was suggested, or close to it, and you watch the number and you adjust and you try. You cut out the obvious things. The desserts. The sodas. Maybe the bread for a while. You lose a few pounds and then you find them again. You go back to the office and the A1C is a little better or a little worse and the doctor says good or let's adjust and writes another prescription or increases the dose on the one you already have.

And you keep going. Appointment to appointment. Number to number. Year to year.

This is what managing it looks like from the inside. And it is exhausting in a way that is almost impossible to explain to someone who has not lived it. Not because the disease is so physically painful — though it can become that. But because of the particular kind of exhaustion that comes from working hard at something and never winning. From doing everything you were told and still watching the disease advance. From being a responsible, compliant patient and still ending up on a second medication. Then a third. Then insulin.

And somewhere in those years — somewhere between the second medication and the third, or the third and the insulin — something shifts inside you. Something quieter and more damaging than the disease itself.

You stop believing the exit exists.

I have sat across from hundreds of patients in that place.

I know what it looks like. It looks like someone who comes to the appointment but has stopped asking questions. Someone who nods at the explanation of why the A1C went up again, who takes the new prescription without pushing back, who has made a private peace with the idea that this is simply who they are now. A diabetic. Someone who manages it.

I had a patient — I will call her Sandra — a hospital administrator, one of the most organized and disciplined people I have ever met. She had been living with type 2 diabetes for eleven years when she came to see me. Eleven years of appointments.

Eleven years of doing what she was told. She had been on three medications, then two, then three again. Her A1C had ranged from 7.8 to 9.4 over that decade, never once dropping below 7.

She sat across from me and said something I have never forgotten.

"I just need you to help me manage it better."

Not reverse it. Not understand it. Not find out whether there was something more possible. Manage it. Because that was the only word that had ever been offered to her. That was the ceiling she had been handed, and after eleven years, she had stopped looking up.

What she did not know — what no one had ever told her — was that eleven years earlier, on the day she was diagnosed, a different conversation had been possible. A conversation that named what was actually happening in her body, that told her what the science was beginning to show, that offered her not just a prescription but a framework and a genuine possibility.

Nobody had that conversation with her.

So she managed. For eleven years. And she came to me still managing, having quietly surrendered the idea that anything else was available.

That is what the lie does.

It is not a single moment of deception. It is a slow accumulation. It is every appointment that ends with an adjusted dose and no mention of remission. It is every conversation about "keeping your numbers in range" that never asks what it would take to make the range unnecessary. It is every year that passes inside a medical system that was designed to manage chronic disease rather than reverse it, during which the patient quietly absorbs the lesson that the system is teaching, even when no one intends to teach it:

This is the best it gets. Learn to live inside it.

That lesson lands differently for different people. For some it arrives as resignation — a quiet letting go of something they once hoped might be possible. For others it arrives as shame — the private belief that the disease keeps advancing because they are not trying hard enough, not disciplined enough, not good enough at being sick in the right way. For others it arrives as anger — at the system, at their body, at the unfairness of a condition that takes so much and gives back so little.

But for almost everyone it arrives. And once it does, it becomes one of the most powerful forces working against recovery — more powerful, in some ways, than the biology itself. Because you cannot fully commit to a path you do not believe leads anywhere.

This is why I have to name the lie before I give you the framework. Because the framework only works if you believe, even tentatively, even with significant doubt, that the exit might be real.

So let me be very direct with you about what the lie is.

The lie is not that diabetes is serious. It is serious. The lie is not that medication is wrong. For many people, medication is necessary and life- saving. The lie is not even that management is bad. Management kept a lot of people alive while we figured out what was actually possible.

The lie is this:

Management is the only option. The ceiling is fixed. Your body cannot do better than this.

That is the lie. And it is wrong.

The American Diabetes Association — together with the Endocrine Society, the European Association for the Study of Diabetes, and Diabetes UK — published its most rigorous and authoritative criteria yet for the remission of type 2 diabetes.

Not management. Not control. Not stabilization.

Remission.

The ADA defined remission as achieving an A1C below 6.5 percent for at least three months without the use of glucose-lowering medications. And in doing so, the most authoritative body in American diabetes care put in writing what the science had been showing for years but the system had not been telling patients:

The science is clear: type 2 diabetes can be reversed.

The framework to do it is what this book provides.

I sat in my own doctor's office with normalized blood sugar levels, no longer needing the medications I had taken for years. My doctor was surprised. He asked what I had been doing. I walked him through the framework I had built — the dietary changes, the fasting protocol, the behavioral tools, the work I had done on the emotional and environmental forces that had been driving my eating for decades.

He listened. He adjusted my medications. He was impressed.

And he never used the word remission.

Not because he was withholding anything. But because the word had not yet fully entered the clinical vocabulary. Because the training pipeline that produced him — that produced me, that produces most physicians practicing today — was built on a model of diabetes as permanent. And models, once built, do not update themselves overnight just because the evidence has moved.

That gap — between what the science now shows and what most patients are still being told — is the lie this chapter is about.

I want to be careful here, because careful matters.

The medical system is not malicious. Physicians are not withholding the possibility of remission to keep patients dependent on medications. The doctors who told you "we can manage it" were telling you the truth as they understood it. They were doing their jobs inside a system that has profound structural limitations — limitations that have nothing to do with their intelligence or their care for you and everything to do with how that system was built.

The system was not designed to do what needs to be done. A follow-up visit in most endocrinology or primary care practices runs fifteen minutes. In fifteen minutes, a physician reviews labs, adjusts medications, documents for insurance, and moves on. There is little room for the education, the behavior change conversation, or the emotional work that real metabolic intervention requires. The training pipeline did not prepare most physicians for that work either — medical education is built around diagnosis and prescription, not around the lifestyle dimensions of disease. And the reimbursement system rewards procedures and pills, not the hours of support that lasting change actually takes. What came out of that system is what you have been experiencing: a prescription, a follow-up, and a quiet suggestion to eat better and exercise more.

And consider this: most physicians have never seen diabetes remission happen in their own patients. Not because it is impossible — but because without the right framework, the right education, and the right support structure, the rate of meaningful lifestyle-driven reversal is low. You cannot point patients toward an outcome you have never personally witnessed. So the message doesn't change because the results don't change because the approach doesn't change.

This is how a lie survives without anyone deciding to tell it. Not through deception but through structure. Not through malice but through momentum. The system keeps moving in the direction it was built to move, and the patients inside it keep receiving the same message, and the ceiling stays in place — invisible and unchallenged — until someone decides to name it.

So let me tell you what you deserved to hear.

On the day you were diagnosed — or on the day you found out the number had crossed the threshold, or on the morning someone woke you from sleep to tell you the doctor had called — here is what should have been said:

You have type 2 diabetes. This is serious, and it deserves your full attention. But it is not a verdict. It is a diagnosis — and a diagnosis, unlike a verdict, points toward a treatment. Your blood sugar is elevated because of a combination of factors: genetic predisposition, lifestyle patterns, environmental forces, and the accumulated metabolic consequences of years of living in a body that was not getting what it needed. None of that makes you a bad person. None of that makes you weak. It makes you human.

Here is also what is true: the science now shows clearly that type 2 diabetes can go into remission. In a significant number of people who are willing to make meaningful changes to how they eat, how they move, how they manage stress, and how they think about the relationship between their emotions and their behavior — the A1C can normalize, the medications can be reduced, and the disease can become, for all practical purposes, reversed.

You are not condemned. You are at the beginning of a process. And the process works.

That is what you deserved to hear.

I am sorry it took this long to arrive.

There is a difference between knowing and existing.

Knowing that remission is possible does not make it happen. This is the gap that most books about diabetes — and most conversations in most exam rooms — never address. The science tells us what is possible. It does not tell us how to get from where you are to where the science says you can be. It does not account for the fact that you have tried to eat differently before and it didn't hold. It does not explain why knowledge of what you should do and the ability to actually do it are two entirely different things, separated by a distance that cannot be crossed by information alone.

Crossing that distance requires a framework. Not a diet. Not a supplement protocol. Not a meal plan you follow for thirty days and then abandon when real life reasserts itself. A framework — a way of understanding your metabolism, your behavior, your emotional life, and your environment that allows you to design a path forward that actually fits the person you are and the life you are actually living.

That framework is what this book is built to give you.

It begins with your body. Specifically, with understanding what is actually happening inside it — not in the simplified, slightly misleading way that diabetes is often explained to patients, but in the way that genuinely illuminates why your body has been doing what it's been doing and what it actually needs to do something different.

Because your body is not broken. It has never been broken. It has been responding — intelligently, consistently, predictably — to the conditions it has been given. Change the conditions, and the body changes with them.

That is where we go next.

CHAPTER TWO

Your Body Is Not Broken — It's Responding

"The body has already been dealing with it and keeping it normal. The diagnosis is new to you. It is not new to your body."

She was sixty-three years old. Her daughter had come with her to the appointment, as she always did. She was diagnosed with type 2 diabetes over thirty years ago — which means she has been living with this disease for longer than some of my younger patients have been alive. For three decades, she managed. She took her medications. She watched her diet, more or less. She came to her appointments. She did what she was told. And for three decades, the message she received — explicitly or implicitly, from every physician she ever saw — was the same:

This is what your life looks like now. Manage it.

She never questioned it. Why would she? Thirty years of the same message from people with medical degrees is a long time to hold an alternative belief.

The day she came off her last diabetes medication, she walked into my exam room and hugged me.

Not because the number had changed. She had seen numbers change before. She hugged me because of what the number now meant — because of the story it was telling her about her own body that she had never been allowed to believe was possible.

"I never realized," she said, "that I could be off medication with diabetes. That I could eat normally as long as I am mindful."

Thirty years. And nobody had told her.

I think about her whenever I sit down to explain diabetes to a new patient. I think about the thirty years she spent carrying a ceiling that was never real. And I think about how different her journey might have looked if someone had taken the time, early on, to explain not just what diabetes is — but what the body was doing, and why, and what that means about what is actually possible.

That is what this chapter is — the explanation she deserved thirty years ago, and the one you deserve now.

When I was growing up in Brooklyn, there were four of us in that apartment. Four kids, third floor, both parents working. My mother would leave for work in the morning and before she walked out the door she would say the same thing she said every morning.

Clean the house.

And of course we would not clean the house. We were kids. We tore it up. All day. Toys, clothes, shoes, dishes — the whole apartment looked like a tornado had passed through it by the middle of the afternoon.

She never carried a key. So when she got home she had to ring the bell from the street, and someone had to walk down three flights of stairs to let her in. That walk down was the only thing standing between us and being caught.

One of us would go down slowly. The rest of us would move.

By the time she made it up the stairs and through the door, the floors were swept. The dishes were stacked. The toys were gone. The apartment looked like we had been working on it all day.

But she was a mother, and mothers know.

If she opened a closet — stuff fell out. If she looked under a bed — stuff was crammed under there. If she checked a cabinet — the cabinet was the new dumping ground.

The floor was clean. The mess had not gone away. It had been moved.

That is what insulin does in the body of someone living with type 2 diabetes.

When you eat a meal, your blood sugar rises. Your pancreas releases insulin. Insulin's job — and it does it well — is to clean. It lowers the sugar in the blood. The numbers come down. The A1C improves on paper. The doctor looks at the chart and says, we have it under control.

But here is the question almost no one asks.

When insulin lowers the blood sugar, where does it put it?

It does not disappear. It does not evaporate. The body has to put it somewhere. And the somewhere is the liver, where it becomes the fat we now call fatty liver disease. It is the abdomen, where it becomes the visceral fat at the center of metabolic syndrome. It is the blood vessels, where it contributes to high blood pressure and cardiovascular disease. It is, increasingly, the brain, where research suggests insulin dysregulation may be involved in dementia.

The sugar was on the floor. Insulin moved it into the closets.

The numbers got better. The disease did not.

This is the part of diabetes management we do not talk about. We measure the floor. We do not measure the closets. And so a person can spend years getting reports that say under control while the closets quietly fill up with everything insulin has been stuffing away.

There is one more thing about that house that matters here.

Now imagine a different version of that day. Imagine the four of us had been cleaning since morning — really cleaning, all day, without stopping. By the time my mother came home, we would have been dragging. The work would still be happening, but on exhausted legs.

The pancreas does the same thing. The beta cells that make insulin are not designed to keep producing at the volume the modern food environment demands of them. They produce. They produce more. They produce more again. And eventually they slow down. Not because they are broken. Because they are tired. Because nothing in their design accounted for being asked to clean this much for this long.

So when a person finally walks into my office with an A1C of 9, what they are usually looking at is not a body that failed.

They are looking at a cleaning crew that has been working overtime for twenty years and finally cannot keep up.

The crew is not the problem. The crew has been doing its job.

The problem is the mess.

And the mess does not stop because the cleaning gets faster. The mess stops when we stop making so much of it.

With that picture in mind, let me explain what insulin actually is and what it actually does.

Insulin is a hormone produced by the beta cells of your pancreas. Its primary job is to manage the glucose — the sugar — that enters your bloodstream when you eat carbohydrates. When you consume carbohydrates, your digestive system breaks them down into glucose, which passes into your blood. Your blood sugar rises. Your pancreas detects the rise and releases insulin in response.

Think of insulin as a key. Your cells — in your muscles, your liver, your fat tissue — have locks on their doors. Glucose cannot enter those cells without a key. Insulin is that key. When insulin binds to the receptor on the cell surface, the door opens, glucose enters, and your blood sugar comes back down. The glucose is then either used immediately for energy or stored for later — as glycogen in the liver and muscles, or as fat when those stores are full.

In a healthy metabolic system, this process is elegant. You eat. Blood sugar rises. Insulin is released. Glucose enters the cells. Blood sugar returns to normal. Insulin levels fall. The system resets and waits for the next meal.

Insulin also does several other things worth understanding. It tells the liver to stop producing glucose — because when you've just eaten, you don't need the liver adding more sugar to blood that is already rising. It promotes the storage of fat and inhibits its breakdown — which is why chronically elevated insulin makes weight loss so difficult. And it signals the kidneys to retain sodium, which affects blood pressure. Insulin is not just a blood sugar hormone. It is a master metabolic regulator whose fingerprints are on almost every system in your body.

When insulin works the way it was designed to work, it is one of the most precisely engineered systems in human biology. The problem is not insulin itself. The problem is what happens when we ask it to do too much for too long.

Here is how I explain diabetes.

Diabetes is a gap.

Specifically, it is the gap between what the body is able to do and what the blood sugar is demanding that it do. Let me show you what I mean.

Imagine your body has the capacity to manage a blood sugar of 150. If your blood sugar is 149, your body handles it. No problem. No diabetes. Now imagine your blood sugar reaches 151. That one point — that single unit of glucose above what your system can currently manage — is the gap. That is where diabetes lives. Not in a dramatic collapse. In a gap.

And here is the part that most patients have never heard:

Your body has been closing that gap for years.

We know from research that by the time someone receives a diabetes diagnosis, their blood sugars have been elevated — or on the verge of elevation — for quite some time. Years, in many cases. But here is why you didn't know: your body was fixing it. Quietly. Continuously. Without asking for your help or your awareness. Your pancreas was working overtime, releasing more and more insulin to keep the blood sugar in a range that looked normal on a lab test. Your body was not failing. It was compensating.

The diagnosis is new to you. It was not new to your body. Your body had already been dealing with this and keeping it normal for longer than you know. The moment that diabetes shows up on a lab result is the moment your body's ability to keep closing that gap finally becomes less than the weight of the gap itself — the amount of glucose being brought in through food, produced by the liver, or sitting unused in the bloodstream because the cells have stopped responding normally to insulin's signal.

That is not failure. That is a body that fought as long as it could and finally needed help.

So what happened to the lock and key system?

Here is the best analogy I know for insulin resistance. Imagine a smoke alarm in your kitchen. The first time it goes off, you pay attention. You investigate. You deal with whatever is causing the smoke. But if that alarm goes off every single day — if it becomes background noise in your home — you start to ignore it. Not because something is wrong with you. Because that is what any nervous system does when a signal becomes constant: it turns down its sensitivity to that signal.

Your cells do the same thing with insulin.

When insulin is chronically elevated — because you are eating in a way that keeps blood sugar and therefore insulin constantly high — your cells begin to downregulate their response. The receptors on the cell surface become less sensitive. The doors become harder to open. Insulin shows up with the key, but the lock has changed. The cell is no longer responding the way it should. This is insulin resistance: the key still exists, but it no longer turns the lock efficiently.

The pancreas, detecting that blood sugar is not coming down the way it should, responds by releasing more insulin. More keys for the stubborn locks. And for a while — sometimes for years — this works. The extra insulin overcomes the resistance. Blood sugar stays in a normal or near-normal range. The lab tests look acceptable. But underneath the surface, the system is under increasing strain.

Eventually, the beta cells of the pancreas — the cells that produce insulin — begin to fatigue under the demand of constant overproduction. Their capacity diminishes. And when the insulin they can produce is no longer enough to overcome the resistance the cells have developed, the gap opens. Blood sugar rises. The lab result changes. And you sit in a doctor's office receiving news that your body has been quietly managing toward for years.

This is the progression of type 2 diabetes. And I want you to notice something important about it: at every stage, the body was doing exactly what a well-designed system does. It was adapting. It was compensating. It was trying to maintain equilibrium under conditions that were working against it. The body did not turn against you. The body was fighting for you, with the tools it had, against conditions that eventually exceeded its capacity to compensate alone.

I want to stay here for a moment, because this is the piece that changes everything.

Insulin resistance is not a malfunction. It is an adaptation.

This is a protective mechanism designed into the body. The ability to downregulate insulin sensitivity protects cells from overstimulation when insulin is chronically elevated. The problem is not that this mechanism exists. The problem is that we now live in an environment that activates it relentlessly — an environment of processed foods engineered to maximize glucose response, of chronic stress that raises blood sugar through cortisol, of sleep deprivation that disrupts insulin signaling, of sedentary patterns that reduce the muscles' ability to take up glucose without insulin's help.

Your body was not designed for this environment. No human body was. And when a system designed for one set of conditions is placed in a fundamentally different set of conditions for long enough, the adaptations that once protected it become the source of the problem.

This is not a character flaw. This is not evidence of weakness or poor discipline or a fundamental inadequacy in you as a person. This is biology responding to conditions. And the single most important implication of that fact is this:

Change the conditions, and the biology changes with them.

Sandra had been told none of this. Thirty years of appointments, and no one had ever explained that her body had been fighting for her — not against her.

Insulin resistance is not a permanent state. It developed in response to conditions over time, and it can be reversed in response to different conditions over time. The cells that stopped listening can learn to listen again. The pancreas that has been overworked can recover function when the demand on it is reduced. The gap that defines diabetes can be closed — not by forcing the body to do something it cannot do, but by changing what we are asking it to respond to.

There is one more consequence of this cellular blockade worth naming, because it explains something my patients struggle with long before they understand the mechanism: when your cells cannot access the glucose in your bloodstream, they generate a starvation signal. And that signal produces real, physiological hunger — regardless of how much energy your body is carrying in storage. The hunger is not a character flaw. It is a symptom.

Your body is not broken. It never was. It has been responding — intelligently, consistently, and in the only direction available to it given what it was being given. What changes now is what we give it.

But before we get to what changes, we need to be honest about what created the conditions in the first place.

Because insulin resistance does not develop in a vacuum. It develops in a life.

The food environment is a significant part of the story. We live surrounded by foods that are specifically engineered to produce rapid, large glucose responses — ultra-processed products designed by food scientists to hit what the industry calls the "bliss point," the precise combination of sugar, salt, and fat that overrides your body's natural satiety signals and keeps you eating past the point of genuine hunger. These foods are cheap, convenient, heavily marketed, and everywhere. Navigating them requires active effort in a way that eating whole, unprocessed foods simply did not for most of human history.

Stress is another part of the story that almost never gets the attention it deserves. When you are under stress — physical, emotional, relational, financial, professional — your body releases cortisol. Cortisol is a hormone designed for short-term emergency response. Among its many functions, it raises blood sugar by prompting the liver to release stored glucose, ensuring you have fuel available for the threat your nervous system believes you are facing. Under chronic stress — which is the kind most of us are actually living with — cortisol remains chronically elevated. Which means blood sugar remains chronically elevated. Which means insulin remains chronically elevated. Which accelerates insulin resistance.

Sleep deprivation compounds everything. A single night of poor sleep measurably reduces insulin sensitivity — the cells become less responsive to insulin's signal after just one disrupted night. Chronic sleep deprivation produces a state of metabolic stress that mimics, in many ways, the trajectory toward type 2 diabetes. And yet sleep is almost never addressed in a standard diabetes management visit.

And then there are the emotional forces — the relationship between how we feel and what we eat, the habits of using food to manage emotions that have been building since childhood, the way that stress and loneliness and boredom and frustration find their way to the kitchen or the drive-through or the bottom of the bag in ways that have nothing to do with physical hunger. This is not weakness. This is neuroscience. And we will come back to it in depth, because it is one of the most important — and most overlooked — dimensions of metabolic health.

All of these forces — the food environment, the stress, the sleep, the emotional relationship with eating — create the conditions that the body responds to. They are not excuses. They are the actual terrain. And you cannot navigate terrain you haven't honestly mapped.

Let me tell you about the sandwich.

Early in my own journey — before my rhythms had stabilized, before I had the language for what I was building — I decided to wear a continuous glucose monitor. Not as a clinical experiment. Not to collect data the way a researcher would. But because I wanted to see myself with the same honesty I was asking of my patients. A CGM is a small sensor that sits just under the skin and measures blood glucose in real time, every few minutes, all day and all night. It is, as I described it then, like putting a mirror on your arm that refuses to lie.

One afternoon during a long clinic day, I grabbed a meal I knew was not ideal. Not balanced. Not strategic. Just convenient – a sandwich that I had eaten before and that I knew, based on its composition and my experience with my own glucose patterns, should send my blood sugar climbing into the upper 180s or touching 200. I ate it quickly between tasks and drove home, already mentally preparing for the spike I expected to see on the monitor.

When I checked the monitor later, my glucose had peaked at 120.

I stared at the number.

Not because of what I had eaten. The food was the same. Not because of some special moment of discipline or intention. I had eaten quickly, distracted, between obligations. Something else had happened. Something upstream of the meal had changed the metabolic context in which the meal landed.

I traced back through the day. And I found it.

Earlier that day, I had walked. Not a workout. Not a structured exercise session. An almost absentminded walk – the kind you do when the destination is close enough to drive but you decide not to. Ten minutes, maybe fifteen. Unhurried. Unremarkable. And it had changed everything about how my body responded to the meal that came hours later.

Here is the biology of what happened. When skeletal muscle contracts during movement, it can take up glucose from the bloodstream independently of insulin – through a separate mechanism that does not require the key to open the lock, because the door opens from the inside. That walk had primed my muscles to absorb glucose more efficiently. So when the sandwich arrived and blood sugar began to rise, the muscles were ready and responsive in a way they would not have been had I sat at my desk all day.

A fifteen-minute walk had blunted a glucose spike by sixty to eighty points. Not because the food changed. Not because of willpower or intention or discipline. Because of one small upstream decision that changed the metabolic conditions in which everything else happened.

That is the body responding. That is the body doing exactly what it was designed to do when given conditions that support it. And that one moment, watching a number on a monitor that should have been 190 sitting quietly at 120, taught me more about the responsiveness of the metabolic system than any textbook had.

The woman who had been coming to see me for years, always with her daughter, who hugged me — she spent thirty years believing the ceiling was fixed.

She wasn't wrong to believe it. She had been given no reason to believe otherwise. Every appointment, every prescription, every follow-up reinforced the same story: manage it. Stay stable. This is your life now.

What changed was not her body. Her body had always been capable of responding differently. What changed was the conditions she was giving it — and the framework she was using to create those conditions consistently, day after day, until the gap that had defined her diabetes for three decades finally closed.

This is the truth that every person with type 2 diabetes deserves to understand before anything else:

The body that developed insulin resistance can reverse insulin resistance. The same responsiveness that created the problem is the responsiveness that solves it.

This is not a promise that it will be easy. It will require consistent effort, a framework that addresses the whole picture — the metabolic, the behavioral, the emotional, the environmental — and the willingness to do something that may feel unfamiliar: trust a body you have been taught to see as the problem.

Your body is not the problem. Your body is the solution — waiting for the right conditions to demonstrate what it has always been capable of.

But before we can change the conditions, we need to understand the forces that have been shaping them. Because the conditions that created your insulin resistance did not arise from food alone. They arose from something deeper — from four powerful forces that have been driving your relationship with eating in ways you may have never fully seen.

That is where we go next.

CHAPTER THREE

The Four Forces — Why You Eat the Way You Eat

The Four Forces

"When we get triggered, we are no longer living in that moment. We are living based on history."

For years, I had a problem I could not explain.

I was an endocrinologist. I understood metabolism. I spent most of my days explaining to patients exactly what was driving their high blood sugars and exactly what they needed to do to bring those numbers down. I had the knowledge. I had the training. I had, if anything, more information about this disease than almost anyone in the room.

And I still couldn't translate that knowledge into better numbers for myself.

The food was driving my blood sugar. That part was clear. If I didn't eat the things that spiked my glucose, my numbers were good. Simple. Logical. Completely obvious to me as a physician.

So why, if I knew what was causing the blood sugar and I knew what was causing the cause, did that knowledge not translate into action?

I started asking my patients the same question — not in those terms, but in the terms of their own lives. Not "what are you eating" but "why are you eating it." Not "don't you know what that does to your blood sugar" but "tell me the story of that food."

What came back changed everything I thought I understood about why people eat the way they eat.

She came in almost panicking.

Easter was coming, and she was already anxious about it. Not because of family obligations or travel plans. Because of the chocolate eggs.

She loved these particular chocolate eggs — a seasonal candy that only appeared around Easter. She couldn't get enough of them. Every year when Easter approached, she would go to the store and buy as many as she could find, then store them throughout the year. She was a woman with diabetes, sitting across from her endocrinologist, telling me she was stockpiling Easter candy. And she knew it was a problem. That wasn't the issue. The issue was that knowing it was a problem had never once stopped her from doing it.

I asked her the question I had started asking my patients when the standard questions weren't getting us anywhere:

"When was the first time you had these chocolate eggs?"

She paused. And then she told me the story.

Her father had been in the military. They moved constantly — new town after new town, always the new kid, never settled, never quite belonging anywhere. And because they were often in smaller communities and her parents were cautious, she was rarely allowed to go to the store by herself. Freedom, in the way most children experience it, was something she watched from a distance.

Then they moved to a town where there was a store just a short distance from their house. And one day, her mother stood on the porch, looked down the street, and said: "You're old enough now. The store is close enough. Go."

She walked down to that store alone for the first time in her life. She was a little girl. Her mother watched from the porch. And when she walked through the door, the man behind the counter sold her these chocolate eggs.

She was in her sixties when she told me this story. The store was gone, her parents were gone, that little girl was now a woman managing a chronic disease. But every Easter, when those chocolate eggs appeared on the shelves, she wasn't buying candy.

She was buying freedom. She was buying autonomy. She was buying the trust her mother placed in her that afternoon when she watched her walk down to the store alone for the first time. She was buying the feeling of that moment — and she had been buying it, every single year, without ever knowing that was what she was doing.

She wasn't eating chocolate eggs. She was eating a memory.

She was not alone.

I had a gentleman who couldn't stop eating a particular candy bar. He knew it was doing damage. He didn't understand why he couldn't stop. When we dug into his story, it turned out that his parents had not been able to care for him and had sent him to live with an uncle. The uncle traveled for work. And every time the uncle came home, he would bring these candy bars as a treat — a signal that he had returned, that he was present, that the boy mattered enough to be thought of.

Every candy bar was his uncle coming home.

I had a patient who couldn't get enough apple pie — not any apple pie, but a specific kind, made a specific way. When we traced it back, it turned out she had not spent much time with her grandmother growing up. But when she did visit, the thing they did together was make apple pies. Every slice was her grandmother's kitchen. Every bite was time she could not get back.

And then there was the patient who could not stop eating oatmeal raisin cookies.

She said she loved them. Could not get enough of them. She would buy a bag, tell herself she was going to have just a few, and find herself at the bottom of the bag before she had made any conscious decision to keep eating. She knew they were raising her blood sugar. She knew she needed to stop. And she could not stop.

I asked her the question.

"When was the first time you loved oatmeal raisin cookies? Where does this start?"

She thought about it for a long moment. And then she said: Sunday mornings.

She had grown up in a household where Sunday had a specific ritual. Every Sunday morning without exception, her mother made oatmeal on the stove — the old-fashioned kind, the kind that takes time, that fills the kitchen with a smell that is warm and slightly sweet and entirely specific to that particular moment of the week. Not the quick oats, not the packets. The real thing, stirred slowly, with milk and a little brown sugar, served in the bowls they only used on Sunday.

And alongside the oatmeal there was toast — the only day of the week they had toast — and glasses of cold milk. The whole family at the table. Unhurried. Together. And then they would get dressed and go to church.

That Sunday morning ritual was safety. It was belonging. It was the weekly proof that the family was whole and together and that the week ahead, whatever it held, would be navigated from a solid foundation.

She did not remember exactly when raisins entered her awareness — somewhere in childhood, raisins became associated with goodness, with health, with the kind of sweet thing her parents approved of. And then one day, she discovered that someone had made a cookie that combined oatmeal and raisins. She remembered the feeling of that discovery. The delight of finding that two things she loved — one because of Sunday mornings, one because of some earlier association she could no longer fully trace — had been combined into a single thing.

She had been eating that discovery ever since.

When she sat in front of the bag of oatmeal raisin cookies, she was not eating a cookie. She was eating Sunday morning. She was eating the smell of oatmeal on the stove and the sound of her family at the table and the warmth of a home that was reliable and safe. She was eating the particular joy of being a child who found something delightful in the world.

She was eating three or four different memories simultaneously, compressed into a single food that had carried all of them for decades without her ever being aware of the cargo it was holding.

That is the taste force at its most complex. Not one memory — a whole architecture of memory. A ritual, a season, a feeling, a discovery, all collapsed into something you can hold in your hand and eat in thirty seconds. And the eating never quite delivers what it promises, because what it promises is a Sunday morning that no longer exists. But the brain keeps reaching for it anyway, because the taste is the closest available portal.

And then there is my own story.

Every time I go back to New York, I have to get pizza, a hot dog, and Chinese food. Always those three. Always in that order, more or less. For years I couldn't explain it — it was just what I did when I was in the city, a ritual I had never examined. Until I did examine it. Until I let myself trace it back.

That was what my father used to get me.

He has been gone for several years now. And every time I land in New York and find myself moving toward those same foods, I am not hungry for pizza, a hot dog, and Chinese food. I am hungry for my father. I am reaching for a feeling I cannot have any other way.

These stories — my patients' and my own — are what gave birth to the H.E.A.T. model. Not a theory I read in a textbook. A pattern I kept seeing in exam room after exam room, conversation after conversation, until it became impossible to ignore.

The H.E.A.T. model identifies four forces that drive non-hunger eating.

H — Habit

E — Emotion

A — Access

T — Taste

These are not the reasons you overeat. They are the reasons you eat when you are not hungry, when you said you wouldn't, when you knew better, when the decision you made in the morning dissolved by the afternoon. They are the triggers. And when a trigger fires, you are no longer making a decision based on the present moment. You are responding to the past.

Let's look at each one.

H — Habit

Habit is eating that has nothing to do with hunger and everything to do with pattern.

You go to the movies, and you get popcorn. Not because you're hungry. Because you go to the movies and you get popcorn. That is what happens at the movies. The two things are linked in your nervous system at a level that precedes conscious decision-making. The environment triggers the behavior before your thinking brain has had a chance to weigh in.

Someone comes to visit and you offer them coffee and a muffin. You get up from your desk to walk to the bathroom and pass a colleague's desk where there is a bowl of candy — and your hand moves toward it before you have made any decision to eat. You finish dinner and move to the couch and find yourself reaching for something sweet, not because dinner was unsatisfying but because that is what happens after dinner on the couch.

The brain uses approximately twenty percent of the body's total energy, and it is relentlessly focused on conserving it. Habits are how it does that — by automating repeated behaviors so they no longer require conscious deliberation. Once a behavior has been repeated enough times in a consistent context, the brain bundles the context and the behavior together and stops asking you to decide. It just does it.

This is brilliant engineering for most of life. It is a significant problem when the automated behavior is one that raises your blood sugar.

The habit force is operating constantly, in the background, linking environments and behaviors in ways you have likely never examined. And what you cannot see, you cannot change.

E — Emotion

Emotion is the force that overrides every decision you have ever made.

I want you to picture a roller coaster. The car starts at the bottom and begins to climb. Slowly at first, then faster. You are holding on. The track curves and rises and you are going up, up, up toward the peak. And at the top of that peak — right at the pinnacle, where you can see everything — you could decide, if you wanted, that you are not going down the other side. You could make that decision clearly and firmly and with complete conviction.

But you are going down the other side.

That is emotion. When anger, frustration, loneliness, boredom, anxiety, grief, or exhaustion climbs high enough, it pushes through any decision you have made about what you will or will not eat. Not because you are weak. Because the emotional brain is physiologically more powerful than the decision-making brain in those moments.

This is why telling yourself "I'm not going to eat that" on a calm Tuesday morning often fails by Thursday afternoon when the meeting went badly and the commute was long and you are tired in a way that sleep doesn't quite fix. The decision was made by one version of your nervous system and is being tested by a completely different version — one that is under load, running on cortisol, and very interested in the fastest available source of relief.

Food is one of the fastest available sources of relief the human brain knows. It produces dopamine. It lowers cortisol temporarily. It works — in the short term. And the brain, under emotional load, is not thinking about the long term. It is thinking about right now.

Emotion is not an excuse. It is an explanation. And it is one of the most important things to understand about your own eating, because until you see the emotion underneath the behavior, you will keep trying to change the behavior while leaving the emotion untouched — and wonder why nothing holds.

A — Access

Access is the simplest force in the H.E.A.T. model, and the most underestimated.

Here is the reality: if you were frustrated or angry or anxious and there was absolutely nothing in your house to eat — no chips in the pantry, no ice cream in the freezer, no leftover anything in the refrigerator — you would have to make an active decision to go get something. You would have to put on shoes. Get in the car. Drive somewhere. Find parking. Walk into a store. Navigate choices. Stand in a line. That is a lot of friction between the emotion and the eating. And friction, in those moments, saves you.

But when the chips are on the counter and the ice cream is in the freezer and the leftover cake is on the second shelf exactly where you put it — the friction disappears. The distance between the impulse and the action collapses to zero. Your hand moves. The package opens. You are eating before the decision has fully formed.

Access is not just about what is in your house. It is about what is on your desk, what is in the break room, what the gas station sells at the register, what sits in a bowl at your colleague's workstation, what is offered at every meeting and every celebration and every moment of transition in your day. We live in an environment of extraordinary food access — cheap, convenient, high-calorie food available at virtually every point in the day, placed specifically to capture the impulsive reach.

You cannot out-discipline access. You can only redesign it.

T — Taste

Taste is the most misunderstood force in the model — and the one with two distinct dimensions that operate very differently from each other.

The first dimension is the one the patient stories have been telling all along.

Taste is memory with a flavor.

The chocolate eggs were not about chocolate. The candy bars were not about sugar. The apple pie was not about apples. The oatmeal raisin cookies were not about oatmeal or raisins. Every food in those stories carried a meaning that had been assigned to it in a specific moment, with a specific person, under a specific emotional condition — and that meaning had been stored alongside the taste in the memory system in a way that made them inseparable. The taste became a portal. A way of going back.

The neuroscience of this is not metaphorical. Taste and smell are the senses most directly connected to the memory and emotion centers of the brain. The olfactory bulb — which processes smell, closely intertwined with taste — has direct anatomical connections to the hippocampus, where memories are formed, and the amygdala, where emotions are processed. This is why a smell can transport you to a specific moment from thirty years ago with a vividness that a photograph cannot match. And it is why a taste can do the same thing — and bring with it not just the memory but the entire emotional state associated with it.

When that woman bought her chocolate eggs, she was not experiencing the taste of chocolate. She was experiencing the taste of freedom. When the patient ate her oatmeal raisin cookies, she was not experiencing the taste of oats and sugar. She was experiencing the taste of Sunday morning — the smell of something warm on the stove, the family at the table, the particular safety of a childhood ritual that told her the world was reliable.

This is one reason why "just eat better" is profoundly incomplete advice. It is addressing the surface of a system that runs much, much deeper.

But there is a second dimension of the Taste force that is not personal at all. It was not formed in your childhood or tied to a specific memory or rooted in a relationship you were trying to hold onto.

It was designed in a laboratory.

In the 1970s, a food scientist and psychophysicist named Howard Moskowitz made a discovery that transformed the processed food industry. Through extensive research and consumer testing, he identified what he called the bliss point — the precise combination of sugar, salt, and fat that produces the maximum pleasure response in the human brain. Not just good taste. Optimized taste. The exact ratio at which the brain's reward system fires most powerfully and drives the strongest desire to repeat the experience.

Once the formula was known, every major food company applied it. Chips, cereals, cookies, sauces, snack foods, beverages — each one engineered not merely to taste good but to hit the neurological sweet spot that overrides satiety and produces the compulsion to keep eating.

Here is the most important clinical detail about how the bliss point works: the food is engineered to produce a short-term pleasure surge and then fade just quickly enough that the brain registers incomplete satisfaction and reaches for more. The goal is not your pleasure. The goal is your return.

When a patient tells me they cannot stop eating a certain food — that they know it is working against their health but they cannot seem to leave it alone — the standard clinical response has historically been some variation of discipline. But when the food has been engineered by teams of food scientists, tested on thousands of consumers, and optimized specifically to override the satiety signals that would otherwise tell you to stop — the problem is not insufficient willpower.

You are not weak. You were targeted.

This does not remove personal agency. You still make choices. The framework in this book is built on the belief that those choices matter. But making better choices requires understanding what you are actually up against — not just your own emotional history and habits, but a food environment that has been deliberately engineered to take advantage of every one of the H.E.A.T. forces simultaneously.

I want to add one more dimension to the Taste and Emotion forces that I have never seen articulated in any clinical framework — but that I have heard described by patients more times than I can count.

Food is not only a source of comfort. For many people, it is a source of company.

One of my patients put it to me in a way that I have thought about many times since. She said that she calls her friends, she calls her family, but they have their own lives. They are not always available. They get tired. They cannot always be what she needs them to be in a particular moment.

"Food is a constant, willing, non-complaining companion. It is always available. I have never gone to food and had it say it doesn't have time right now. It never cries at me. It never says it's too busy. It's always there, always willing, always the same."

She was not describing gluttony. She was describing loneliness. She was describing the way that food fills a relational space when the human relationships in our lives are temporarily unavailable, insufficient, or complicated in ways that food simply is not.

This is also why food is often treated as a reward — as compensation earned by having been good or productive or disciplined. The problem with food-as- reward is that it creates a pressure and a tension around the food that does not exist when food is simply food. I try to help patients separate these two things: to eat the food because they want the food. Not because they earned it. Not because it is the only friend available. Not because they are trying to go back to a Sunday morning that no longer exists.

So here is what the H.E.A.T. model is really saying.

You are not eating because you are hungry. You are eating because you are triggered. Whether it is the habit cue of sitting down to watch television, the emotional surge of a difficult conversation, the frictionless access of food sitting within arm's reach, the taste memory of a moment you are trying to return to, or the bliss-point engineering of a food designed to override your satiety signals — you are no longer making a decision in the present. You are responding to something deeper.

This is not a moral failing. This is the ordinary functioning of a human nervous system shaped by decades of experience, living in an environment designed to exploit every one of these forces simultaneously.

And here is why it matters so much for your diabetes specifically: every time the H.E.A.T. forces drive you to eat in ways that spike your glucose, you are generating the exact metabolic conditions that sustain and deepen insulin resistance. Each force, individually, creates a glucose event. Collectively, sustained over weeks and months and years, they create the pattern that defines metabolic disease.

This is why managing diabetes is not primarily about knowing what to eat. It is about understanding what is driving you to eat what you eat. Without that understanding, you are treating the surface of a system that runs from the bottom up.

When the H.E.A.T. model finally crystallized for me — when I looked at all of those patient stories and all of my own and saw the pattern underneath them — it felt like a light coming on in a dark room.

Not because it was complicated. Because it was true. Because it explained, in plain terms, something that years of standard dietary advice had never been able to explain: why intelligent, motivated, informed people — people who knew exactly what they should do — kept not doing it.

The knowledge was never the problem. The H.E.A.T. forces were the problem. And they were operating underneath the level at which most dietary advice is aimed.

When I started sharing this framework with patients — when I started asking them not what they were eating but why, and helping them trace the habit, the emotion, the access, the taste memory, and the engineered craving — something shifted in those exam room conversations. People stopped defending themselves and started examining themselves. They stopped arriving with shame and started arriving with curiosity. Because naming the forces gave them something they had never had before:

A way to see what was actually happening.

And what you can see, you can work with.

You now have three things that most people with diabetes were never given.

You know that the exit is real — that diabetes remission is a documented, scientifically validated possibility, not a fantasy.

You know that your body is not broken — that insulin resistance is an adaptation, that the gap can be closed, and that your biology is responsive to the conditions you give it.

And you know why knowledge alone has never been enough — that four powerful forces, including a food environment deliberately engineered to work against your health goals, have been operating underneath your eating behavior in ways that no amount of information could override by itself.

Now we build the three pillars.

The three pillars of The Diabetes Exit address the metabolic conditions that sustain insulin resistance directly and specifically. They are not a diet. They are a design — a way of structuring what you eat, when you eat, and how you think about the relationship between food and your body that creates the conditions for your biology to do what it has always been capable of doing.

The first pillar is where everything else begins.

A few years ago we were putting up Christmas lights at the house.

I want to set the scene because the scene matters. There is a holly bush outside our home — at least, my wife says it is a holly bush, and I have never argued the point. My job in our house, every December, is the same job most husbands have. Get the lights out of the storage box. Untangle them. Put them up.

So I was walking from the storage closet toward the front of the house with an armful of lights. I had no plan. I was not heading anywhere specific. I was just walking, the way you walk when you are halfway through a chore and your brain is already on the next thing.

And my wife stepped out of the front door.

She looked at me. She looked at the lights. She looked at the holly bush. And she said:

Don't put any lights on my holly bush.

I want you to understand something. I had not been planning to put lights on the holly bush. The thought had never entered my mind. The bush was not on the route. The bush was not in my consciousness. I was a man walking past a bush with lights in his arms.

But the second she said don't — something in my brain woke up.

The first thing I thought was: wait a minute. Whose holly bush is this? She said her holly bush. It is not her holly bush. It could be my holly bush. It could be our holly bush. But it is not her holly bush.

Then I thought: maybe lights would actually look good on the holly bush.

Then I thought: I should get the ladder.

So I went and got the ladder. And I went back and got more lights. And I started walking toward the bush.

She watched the whole thing.

And as I was setting up, she came over, and she put her hand on my arm, and she said — very sweetly:

Honey. Thank you for putting the lights up.

I knew what she was doing. I could feel it happening in real time. I knew it was reverse psychology. I knew she was redirecting me. And I knew I was going to fold.

I took the ladder down. I took the lights down. I put everything back in the garage.

That is reactance.

It is one of the most well-documented principles in human psychology. When you tell someone don't, something in the brain registers it as a threat to their freedom. And the way the brain protects freedom is by leaning toward the forbidden thing, not away from it. The prohibition itself creates the pull. Not the thing. The prohibition.

Now think about how that plays out in the life of a person who has been told, since the day they were diagnosed:

Don't eat sugar. Don't eat bread. Don't eat rice. Don't eat fruit. Don't eat at night. Don't eat that. Don't eat this. Don't.

Every don't is a holly bush.

Every prohibition wakes up the same circuitry that woke up in me when my wife said her holly bush. The food becomes more interesting. The restriction becomes more present. The willpower battle gets bigger, not smaller, every time someone tries to fight harder against it.

This is why diet protocols built on don't almost always fail in the long run. It is not because the patient is weak. It is because the framing itself is fueling the very behavior the patient is trying to extinguish.

The Diabetes Exit is not built on don't.

It is built on understanding what is driving the eating in the first place — the H, the E, the A, the T — and changing the conditions so that the food no longer carries the meaning it has been carrying. When the meaning changes, the pull changes. The brain does not have to fight a thing that is no longer asking to be fought.

You cannot will yourself out of reactance. You can only stop creating the conditions that activate it.

PART TWO

The Framework

CHAPTER FOUR

The First Pillar — Decrease Insulin

"It is not the insulin itself that is the problem. It is the excess."

Of the three pillars in this framework, this one comes first because everything else depends on it.

In Chapter Two, we looked at what happens when insulin spends years cleaning a house that keeps getting messier. The floor stays clean. The closets fill. The body hits a point where the cleaning crew, however hardworking, cannot keep up with the mess.

The first pillar is about closing the closets. About reducing what insulin is being asked to manage in the first place, so the system can do less and accomplish more.

It Is Not the Insulin. It Is the Excess.

I want to start this chapter by making a distinction that most diabetes books never make — and one that reframes the entire problem you are trying to solve.

You have heard the term insulin resistance. It is the phrase used most commonly to describe what underlies type 2 diabetes. And while it is not wrong, it points at the wrong place. It implies that the cell is the problem. That something inside you has malfunctioned.

But the cell is not the problem. The cell is responding to the problem.

The more precise term — and the one that points us toward the actual target — is hyperinsulinemia.

Hyper means excess. Insulinemia means insulin in the blood. Hyperinsulinemia is chronically elevated insulin — not insulin doing what insulin is supposed to do, but insulin present at levels above what the body was designed to sustain for extended periods. The amount above and beyond what the body was designed to sustain is the amount that drives the damage.

Let me be clear about what insulin itself does correctly. Insulin regulates blood sugar. It facilitates glucose uptake into cells. It helps the liver store excess glucose as glycogen. It promotes protein synthesis and supports tissue repair. Insulin, at normal physiological levels, is essential. It is not the enemy.

But when insulin is chronically elevated — chronically present above what the body was designed to sustain, day after day, month after month, year after year — it begins to do something very different. Excess insulin stimulates appetite. It drives fat storage, particularly around the abdomen. It raises triglycerides and disrupts cholesterol metabolism. It promotes inflammation. It raises blood pressure. It accelerates the cellular aging process.

Every complication you associate with metabolic disease — the weight that will not move, the blood pressure that keeps climbing, the inflammation that drives fatigue — has hyperinsulinemia somewhere in its origin story. This is why the first pillar is decrease insulin. Address the excess at its source, and the downstream consequences begin to resolve.

The weight that would not move regardless of how hard you tried — hyperinsulinemia was the reason. Not your effort. The hormonal environment your effort was working against.

Two Pictures of the Problem

Before we talk about how to decrease insulin, I want to offer two analogies that I use in my exam room. They have changed how hundreds of my patients understand what is actually happening in their bodies.

The first is the piano.

Imagine you have a grand piano in your living room and you want to move it to another room. You walk up to it and try to lift it. Most of us cannot. We cannot pick up a grand piano. Now here is my question: is there something wrong with you?

The answer is no. There is nothing wrong with you. The piano is simply too heavy for what you are currently capable of lifting. Your muscles are not defective. Your effort is not insufficient. The load just exceeds your current capacity.

That is what is happening with insulin in type 2 diabetes. The insulin is not broken. It is not defective. It is doing exactly what it was designed to do.

But what it is being asked to manage — the glucose load, the chronic excess of sugar in the blood — has become too heavy for the amount of insulin the body can produce.

Now here is the beautiful implication of this analogy. What if the piano got lighter? What if someone sprinkled something on it that reduced its weight? If somehow the load became lighter, the same amount of insulin — without any change to the insulin itself — could suddenly handle the job. Not because anything changed in the mechanism. Because what it was being asked to carry changed.

This is what decreasing insulin is about. Not replacing the insulin or forcing the pancreas to produce more. Making the load lighter so the insulin the body already has can do its job effectively. When we reduce the refined carbohydrates that spike glucose, when we give the system consistent recovery time, when we move our bodies so that muscles absorb glucose independently of insulin — we are making the piano lighter. The same insulin accomplishes more because there is less for it to carry.

The second analogy is the suitcase.

Most people have heard the lock-and-key model of insulin: insulin is the key, and the cell has a lock on its door. When insulin fits the lock, the door opens and glucose enters, and insulin opens the door to let glucose in. This model is useful but incomplete. It implies that the only reason glucose cannot get into the cell is that the door is stuck. That insulin is failing to unlock it.

But there is another possibility entirely. What if the door can open — but the cell is already full?

Think about packing a suitcase for a trip. You pack everything you need. Then a travel companion asks if you can fit one more thing. You open the suitcase, manage to squeeze it in, close it carefully. Then another companion asks for the same. You open it, sit on it to close it, manage. Now a third person asks. You open the suitcase and try — but nothing else is going in. Not because the suitcase is broken. Because it is already packed.

Research now suggests that a significant part of what we call insulin resistance operates exactly this way. The cells — particularly muscle cells — become infiltrated with fat. Not necessarily because the person is obese on the outside, but because excess fat has accumulated inside the cellular machinery and left no room for glucose to enter. Insulin shows up with the key, the door opens, and the glucose cannot get in because the cell is already at capacity.

The implication for treatment is important. We are not just trying to fix the key or repair the lock. We are trying to empty the suitcase. When body fat decreases, when the fat that has infiltrated the cells is metabolized, space opens up. And when that space opens, the insulin that has been struggling to do its job can suddenly do it — because the obstacle was never the mechanism. It was the luggage.

Both of these analogies point toward the same truth: the problem is rarely the insulin itself. The problem is what the insulin is being asked to manage, and what it has been trying to store. Change those conditions, and the insulin works.

Three Ways to Decrease Insulin

There are three primary ways to decrease insulin, and they work best in combination.

The first is to reduce the inputs that drive insulin production — specifically, the refined carbohydrates and added sugars that produce rapid, large glucose spikes and therefore demand large insulin responses.

The second is to give the system recovery time through structured fasting — periods without food during which insulin levels fall, the cells restore their sensitivity, and the body shifts from storage mode to release mode.

The third — and one that most conversations about insulin never mention — is to help your body use the insulin it already has more efficiently. This is where movement becomes metabolically profound in a way that goes far beyond burning calories.

Remember the sandwich from Chapter Two.

I wore a continuous glucose monitor and ate a meal that should have pushed my blood sugar into the 180s — only to watch it peak at 120. The difference was a walk I had taken earlier that day. Unhurried. Unremarkable. Maybe fifteen minutes.

When skeletal muscles contract during movement, they activate a pathway that allows them to take up glucose directly from the bloodstream — independently of insulin. The mechanism involves GLUT4 transporters activated through a process that does not require insulin's key to open the cell door, because during exercise, the door opens from the inside. The contracting muscle bypasses the insulin system entirely.

What this means practically is that when you move, your muscles take on some of the glucose burden that would otherwise require insulin to manage. The insulin already circulating gets to focus on the remaining load rather than being overwhelmed by the full demand. The system becomes more efficient. And over time, as this mechanism is activated regularly, insulin sensitivity improves — not just in the moment of movement, but in the hours and days that follow.

This is why a fifteen-minute walk is not just about burning calories. It activates a metabolic pathway that changes how your body handles glucose for hours afterward. The energy expenditure is not the therapeutic mechanism. The insulin efficiency is. Strength training amplifies this effect further. When you build metabolically active muscle tissue, you are increasing the size and capacity of the glucose-absorbing system that operates independently of insulin. More muscle means more insulin- independent glucose uptake capacity. More capacity means less demand on the insulin system.

The Carbohydrate Conversation

The carbohydrate conversation is one most people get wrong in both directions.

Carbohydrates are not the enemy.

Uncontrolled carbohydrates are the enemy. There is a significant difference, and getting this wrong in either direction costs you.

If you eliminate all carbohydrates, you eliminate fiber-rich vegetables, legumes, and whole foods that support metabolic health, gut function, and satiety. You make the approach unsustainable, and unsustainable approaches produce the yo-yo pattern that actually worsens insulin resistance over time.

If you eat carbohydrates indiscriminately — refined flour, added sugars, ultra-processed foods engineered for maximum glucose response — you generate the chronic insulin surges that drive hyperinsulinemia and everything that follows.

The goal is quality and quantity. Understanding which carbohydrates work with your metabolism and which ones work against it, and adjusting the balance deliberately.

Refined carbohydrates — white flour, white rice, many packaged breads, pastries, cereals, and anything with added sugar — are processed in ways that remove the fiber and structural components that slow glucose absorption. When you eat them, glucose enters the bloodstream rapidly. The pancreas responds with a large insulin surge. Blood sugar spikes and crashes. The crash drives hunger. Hunger drives eating. Eating drives the next spike. This cycle, repeated across years, is the engine of hyperinsulinemia.

Complex carbohydrates — non-starchy vegetables, legumes, whole grains in their less-processed forms — still contain glucose, but they deliver it slowly. The fiber slows absorption. The glucose enters the bloodstream gradually. The insulin response is smaller and more manageable. The person does not crash and reach for food an hour later.

One of the most valuable things I did during my own reversal journey was wear a continuous glucose monitor and watch what different foods actually did to my blood sugar in real time. Not what the glycemic index table said they should do. What they actually did, in my body, on specific days, under specific conditions. What I found surprised me repeatedly — and taught me more about my own metabolism than any textbook had. This is why I encourage my patients to monitor. The data is not just clinical information. It is a real-time education in how your specific body responds to your specific choices.

The Case for Fasting

Almost every patient I have ever introduced fasting to has said the same thing:

"I can't fast. I have to eat."

I understand why they say it. We have been surrounded our entire lives by messaging that tells us we must eat frequently, that skipping meals is dangerous, that a growling stomach is a medical emergency. Most of this messaging is not based on metabolic science. Much of it was shaped by the food industry, which has a significant financial interest in you eating as frequently as possible.

The body was not designed for a constant fed state. For most of human history, food was not available around the clock. The body developed exquisitely effective mechanisms for operating during periods without food — mechanisms that include accessing stored fat for energy, clearing damaged cellular components through autophagy, restoring insulin sensitivity, and regulating hunger hormones in ways that actually reduce appetite over time.

The growling stomach is not starvation. It is the migrating motor complex — a wave of muscular contractions that sweeps through the digestive system during fasting, clearing undigested food and maintaining gut health. It is the body doing its housekeeping. It is a signal that says stomach is empty — not body is in crisis.

The fear of blood sugar dropping during a fast is legitimate for people on certain medications — particularly insulin or sulfonylureas — and if you are on those medications, fasting requires coordination with your healthcare provider to adjust doses appropriately. For everyone, working with your healthcare provider as you implement any fasting practice is the right approach. Your healthcare provider can monitor your response and adjust your care accordingly.

When you fast, insulin levels fall. Not crash — fall. Gradually and beneficially. And as insulin falls, the metabolic shifts that restore insulin sensitivity begin to occur. The cells that had been tuning out the chronically elevated signal begin to respond again. The fat that had been locked in storage begins to be released for energy. The hunger hormones that had been dysregulated begin to recalibrate. The system starts to heal.

Let me tell you what fasting felt like from the inside.

I had been doing intermittent fasting in various forms for years before I committed to it seriously as part of my reversal process. What changed when I committed more fully was the depth of what I began to experience.

As I extended my fasting periods, something shifted that I had not anticipated. People talk about mental clarity during fasting, and I had been skeptical — as I tend to be skeptical of anything that sounds like it belongs in a wellness magazine. But the clarity arrived. Not dramatically. Just quietly present. A sharpness of thought, an absence of the low-level mental fog that I had normalized without noticing it was there.

The other shift — the one that surprised me most — was what I can only describe as the food noise going away. If you live with diabetes or with hyperinsulinemia or with chronic blood sugar dysregulation, you likely know what food noise is even if you have never used that term. It is the background hum of food-related thoughts that runs constantly — what to eat next, what you should not have eaten, what you are craving, when the next meal is. It is exhausting in a way that is difficult to articulate until it stops.

When I was fasting seriously, the food noise went away. I was not thinking about food constantly. I was not fighting cravings. The silence was remarkable. I began to look forward to fasting. Not as deprivation. As relief.

And then there were the numbers. My A1C, which had spent years in ranges I was ashamed of, began to move. My weight, which had been above 260 for over a decade and had never broken below 200 in fifteen years, began to fall. Then broke through 200. Then kept going.

Fasting was the scalpel. Not the only tool, but the sharpest one.

Where to Start

If you are not fasting at all right now, your first step is to extend the overnight window. Most people already fast for seven or eight hours while they sleep. Simply delay breakfast by one or two hours and you have created a ten-hour fasting window. That is your beginning. It costs nothing. It requires no special equipment. And it begins to lower your baseline insulin in ways that accumulate over time.

If you are on medication for diabetes, you must coordinate any fasting changes with your healthcare provider before you begin. As fasting lowers your blood sugar and your insulin sensitivity improves, the medication doses that were calibrated for your previous metabolic state may become too high. The goal is for your healthcare provider to be reducing your medications as your body gets better. That is a good problem to have. But it needs to be managed carefully.

Walk. Even ten minutes. Even around your living room. The insulin efficiency that movement creates starts with the first step. Not the ten- thousandth step. The first one.

Drink water. This one is remarkably underestimated. Staying well hydrated can meaningfully lower blood sugar levels. When the body is dehydrated, blood becomes more concentrated, which raises the relative concentration of glucose. Hydration dilutes that concentration and supports the kidneys in filtering excess glucose. Starting the day with water before anything else — before coffee, before food, before the phone — is one of the simplest, most overlooked metabolic interventions available to you right now, today, at no cost.

And manage inflammation. Chronic inflammation — from poor sleep, chronic stress, inflammatory foods, or underlying conditions like autoimmune disease — directly worsens insulin resistance. Cortisol rises in inflammatory states and drives blood sugar up independently of what you eat. Anti-inflammatory practices — movement, sleep, stress reduction, and foods rich in omega-3 fatty acids, vitamin D, and turmeric — are not supplements to the framework. They are part of it.

Let me close this chapter with what happens when the first pillar begins to work.

Blood sugar begins to stabilize. The spikes become smaller. The crashes become less pronounced. The baseline begins to drift downward toward a range the body recognizes as manageable.

Weight begins to move. Because insulin is the primary hormone that locks fat in storage, lowering insulin is the prerequisite for meaningful fat loss. People who cut calories without addressing their insulin levels often fail to lose weight because the hormonal environment still says store, not release. Change the hormonal environment first, and the weight follows.

Energy improves. The person who is no longer riding a blood sugar roller coaster through the day has a steadiness of energy that does not depend on the next meal. The peaks and crashes smooth out. The afternoon collapse disappears. The morning heaviness lifts.

Appetite recalibrates. The food noise begins to quiet. Hunger becomes a signal that arrives and departs cleanly, rather than a constant presence demanding attention.

And the A1C — the number that summarizes the last three months of blood sugar management — begins to move in a direction that no one told you was possible.

The woman in her sixties who came off her last diabetes medication after thirty years and walked into my exam room and hugged me — the first pillar was part of what began to lift her ceiling. The same mechanism is available to you.

But decreasing insulin alone is not the complete picture. Because even as insulin levels begin to normalize, the body's appetite signals — which have been dysregulated for years — need their own attention. Hunger is not just a function of blood sugar. It is a hormonal conversation involving multiple systems, and understanding how to participate in that conversation rather than be controlled by it is the work of the second pillar.

That is where we go next.

CHAPTER FIVE

The Second Pillar — Suppress Appetite

"You could decide with your mind that you are not going to eat. But when the hormonal surge happens, you are going to eat."

I have heard some version of this sentence from more patients than I can count.

"If you can just help me not be hungry, I can do the rest."

Not one patient. Dozens. Hundreds, if not thousands. Said in different ways, from different chairs, in different seasons of their lives. But always the same essential confession: the knowledge is not the problem. The discipline is not entirely the problem. The hunger — the relentless, hormonal, seemingly uncontrollable hunger that overrides every decision made in a calm moment — that is the problem.

I understood exactly what they meant. Because I had lived it. I was an endocrinologist with a fellowship in diabetes and metabolism. I knew the science of every hormone involved in appetite regulation. And I was still making peanut butter and jelly sandwiches immediately after finishing a full meal — not because I was hungry, but because my mind was already moving toward the next eating event before the current one had ended.

That is not a willpower problem. It is a biological problem — hormonal in part, behavioral in part, and environmental in part. And it has a solution.

Before we can talk about suppressing appetite, we need to be clear about what appetite actually is — and how it differs from hunger. This distinction is the foundation of everything in this chapter.

Hunger is a physiological need. It is the body saying: I require energy. I need fuel. Hunger does not care what the food looks like. It does not care whether it tastes good or carries pleasant memories or feels a particular way in the mouth. Hunger is a biological signal, regulated by hormones and energy status, that says the body needs calories and nutrients. That is all it is. That is all it cares about.

Appetite is something different. Appetite is a desire — a cognitive event, not a physiological one. Appetite involves memory, anticipation, emotional associations, sensory appeal, and all the psychological and environmental forces we explored in the H.E.A.T. model. Appetite cares very much about what the food tastes like. It cares about the aroma, the texture, the temperature, the specific brand, the memories attached to the experience. It cares whether you are bored or stressed or celebrating or lonely.

Think of it this way. Hunger says: I need food. Any food. Fuel the body. Appetite says: I want that specific thing. The one that feels a certain way. The one that takes me somewhere.

Here is why this distinction matters clinically — and I want to be precise here, because the answer is more complex than most books on this subject acknowledge. In type 2 diabetes, both systems are broken simultaneously. The appetite has been amplified and dysregulated by years of hyperinsulinemia, emotional patterns, environmental cues, and engineered foods. But the hunger itself — the physiological signal that forms the foundation of this distinction — has also been compromised in ways that are documented, measured, and specific to this disease. Before I explain what the second pillar does about it, I want you to understand exactly what you have been dealing with.

You cannot suppress appetite by simply eating less. Eating less addresses hunger — the body's caloric need. But appetite is a brain conversation, not a stomach conversation. You cannot out-restrict the brain. You can only change the conditions under which the brain is operating. And that is exactly what this pillar is designed to do.

Before we go further, I want to name something I wish every physician said aloud to every person with type 2 diabetes at the first appointment.

What you have been experiencing — the constant hunger, the hunger that returns an hour after a full meal, the hunger that never seems to be satisfied — has a medical name. It is called polyphagia. It is listed in clinical textbooks alongside excessive thirst and frequent urination as one of the recognized symptoms of diabetes. The American Diabetes Association recognizes it. Your endocrinologist has a word for it. It is a documented, physiological consequence of how this disease operates in the body.

You were not told this. Most people are never told this. And so you did what any reasonable person does with an unexplained symptom: you decided it was your fault. You called it weakness. You called it a lack of discipline. You measured yourself against it and found yourself lacking, every single time.

You were not lacking. You were symptomatic.

Every patient I have ever said this to has gone quiet for a moment. What you are about to read is why.

The hunger in type 2 diabetes is broken at four simultaneous levels. Each one matters, because each one explains why the hunger feels like something you should be able to overcome — and cannot.

At the first level, your cells are starving. Not because you are not eating. Because the glucose in your bloodstream — the fuel that should be entering your cells to power them — cannot get in. The lock has changed. So your cells send a starvation signal to your brain. And your brain, unable to distinguish between real starvation and metabolic starvation, responds the only way it knows how: it drives you toward food. The tank is full. The gauge reads empty.

At the second level, the hormones that regulate hunger have lost their calibration. Leptin — the signal your fat cells send to tell the brain you have enough energy stored — has been chronically elevated for so long that the brain has stopped listening. The off switch is broken. Ghrelin — the hunger signal produced by your stomach — is supposed to fall reliably after a meal. In metabolic disease, it often does not. The hunger signal stays elevated. The horn gets stuck on. And the GLP-1 that should cascade through the body after eating, slowing digestion and telling the brain the meal is complete — it is markedly reduced in type 2 diabetes, more severely than most patients are ever told.

And that is only two of the four levels operating simultaneously in your body.

At the third level, the hypothalamus — the region of the brain responsible for integrating all of these signals and coordinating the hunger-satiety response — has itself become insulin resistant. The very organ that is supposed to be the command center for this system can no longer read the signals properly. It is not only that the signals are broken. The processor has been compromised by the same disease process driving the blood sugar.

At the fourth level — the one that closes the loop — high blood glucose actively abolishes the sensation of fullness after eating. In measured clinical studies, type 2 diabetic patients report feeling less full after a meal than before it began. The disease inverts the satiety response.

You eat, and the hunger worsens.

That is not a metaphor. That is the measured clinical finding.

All four of these layers are operating simultaneously in a body with type 2 diabetes. That is polyphagia. Not appetite. Not a failure of self-control. A disease state — one that requires a different kind of response than the one you have been trying.

None of this is in your head. All of it has been measured.

There is one more thing you deserve to know. It is the finding that changed how I understand what my patients are up against.

When hunger fires — the kind generated by cellular starvation and stuck ghrelin and failing satiety signals — it does not just make you want food. It changes your brain. Specifically, it impairs the prefrontal cortex: the region responsible for planning, impulse control, and the deliberate decision-making that allows you to choose differently when the craving arrives.

The hunger reduces your capacity for the very thing you are asking yourself to use against it.

It promotes what researchers call future discounting — the state in which an immediate, smaller reward feels more compelling than a larger, delayed one. It weakens the prefrontal cortex's inhibitory control over the amygdala, making emotional responses more intense and food-seeking feel more urgent. The hypothalamic cells that drive hunger are strongly linked to the structure and function of the prefrontal cortex — signaling in one affects the other. What is happening in one affects the other.

This is the full picture of what you have been fighting. Not just the hunger. Not just the hormones. A disease process that generates a relentless biological signal and simultaneously degrades the neural capacity to resist it. These two things do not happen one after another. They happen at the same time, in the same brain, every time the hunger fires.

The solution is not to try harder. It is to change the biological conditions so that the signal is no longer the enemy.

In Chapter Eight, I demonstrate this with a volunteer and twenty dollars. The full exercise lives there, where it belongs. But here is the point it makes: trying to hold back that pull toward food with determination is like trying to hold your breath with money on the table. The mind reaches its limit. The body takes over.

This is what I want family members of people with diabetes to understand — and what I want every person who has ever blamed themselves for not having enough willpower to hear. You are not failing at discipline. You are fighting a hormonal imbalance with a tool — willpower — that was never designed for that fight. The second pillar is not about eating less through greater self-control. It is about restoring the hormonal signals that make appetite manageable in the first place.

My wife has a memory of the early years of our marriage that we still talk about.

We would finish a full meal together — a real meal, a complete dinner, nothing skimped. And before we had even fully cleared the table, I would make myself a peanut butter and jelly sandwich. Not because I was still hungry. Not because the meal had been inadequate. But because my mind was already moving toward the next eating event — already planning, already anticipating, already reaching forward. I had just eaten. And I was already thinking about eating again.

I experienced it as normal — as simply who I was. It did not occur to me that what I was experiencing was not a character trait. It was a hormonal condition.

I have another memory involving juice that captures something different about appetite — its sensory, almost transcendent quality. A friend was visiting and I went to the refrigerator, poured a glass of juice, and started drinking on the way back to the living room. I stopped in the kitchen doorway. Something about it — the sweetness, the cold, the way it felt going down — transported me. I was completely elsewhere for a moment. Fully absorbed.

My friend said to me afterward: I have never seen anyone have that kind of experience with juice.

He was not criticizing me. He was accurately describing what he had witnessed: a person being transported by a sensory experience that had nothing to do with physical hunger. That is the appetite system operating at full power. It is not imagined. It is not weakness. It is the brain doing exactly what years of conditioning have trained it to do. And understanding that is the beginning of being able to work with it rather than be controlled by it.

To understand appetite suppression, you need to understand the hormones that govern hunger. Here are the key players, explained the way I explain them in my exam room.

Ghrelin — The Hunger Hormone

Ghrelin is produced primarily in the stomach and its job is simple: it tells your brain you are hungry. It rises before meals and falls after eating. In a healthy metabolic system, ghrelin rises appropriately when the body genuinely needs fuel and falls reliably after a satisfying meal. The relationship is clean. Eat, feel full, stop being hungry. Wait, feel hungry again. Eat.

In a dysregulated system — one shaped by years of hyperinsulinemia, poor sleep, and chronic stress — ghrelin does not behave this way. It stays elevated longer than it should. It rises at times unrelated to the body's actual energy needs. It responds to emotional cues, environmental triggers, and habitual eating patterns that have nothing to do with the stomach being empty. And because insulin itself stimulates ghrelin, the person with chronically elevated insulin has chronically stimulated hunger — not because the body needs food, but because the hormone system has been set to "hungry" as its default state.

This is why people with metabolic disease often feel hungry shortly after eating. This is why the person who had breakfast two hours ago and is objectively not calorie-deficient finds themselves reaching for something at ten in the morning. The ghrelin signal is not responding to actual energy status. It is responding to a system that has lost its calibration.

Leptin — The Satiety Hormone

Leptin is produced by fat cells and its job is equally simple: it tells your brain you have enough stored energy and do not need to eat more. It is the off switch. When it is working correctly, rising leptin levels signal the hypothalamus to reduce appetite, increase metabolism, and stop the drive to seek food.

Here is the cruel irony of obesity and metabolic disease: people who carry excess body fat have more fat cells, which means they produce more leptin. They are not leptin deficient. They are leptin resistant.

Think of it like the smoke alarm I described when we talked about insulin resistance — the one that goes off so often the family stops hearing it. The same principle applies here. The alarm is still sounding. The signal is still being sent. But the brain has adapted by turning down its sensitivity — because a signal that never stops eventually gets treated as background noise rather than as an alert requiring action. The off switch stops working.

The result is a brain that receives abundant leptin and still interprets the body as starving. It keeps driving hunger. It keeps defending the stored fat as necessary for survival. It keeps making eating feel urgent even when the body has more than enough energy in reserve.

This is not weakness. This is a broken feedback loop. And willpower — the instruction to simply eat less and try harder — is being applied to a system whose fundamental communication mechanism has been compromised. You cannot out-decide a misfiring hypothalamus. The second pillar works not by demanding more discipline from this broken system but by restoring the system's ability to regulate itself.

GLP-1 — The Slow Down Signal

Glucagon-like peptide-1 is released by cells in the intestine in response to eating. It slows gastric emptying — keeping food in the stomach longer, extending the feeling of fullness. It stimulates insulin secretion in a glucose- dependent way, which helps regulate blood sugar after meals. And it acts directly on the brain's appetite centers to reduce hunger.

You may have heard of GLP-1 receptor agonists — medications in this class that have transformed metabolic medicine. These medications work because the GLP-1 pathway is a genuine and powerful appetite regulation mechanism. When it is functioning well, it creates a natural sense of satiety and reduces the urgency of hunger in ways that make portion control feel possible rather than heroic.

The lifestyle practices in this chapter — the foods you eat, the timing of meals, regular movement, the protein intake, the sleep — all support natural GLP-1 function. The medications amplify a pathway the body already has. The framework activates it without medication. Both work toward the same destination. If you are on a GLP-1 medication, the practices in this chapter work alongside it. If you are not, these practices work to activate the same pathway through natural means. The specific mechanism matters here. Protein — particularly protein consumed alongside healthy fat — activates receptors in the gut with high affinity for amino acids, directly stimulating endogenous GLP-1 release. This is one reason that protein and healthy fat at every meal is not only a satiety strategy. It is a GLP-1 activation strategy. The framework creates conditions where the body's own satiety signaling system can function as it was designed — conditions that were not present when hyperglycemia was suppressing that function.

Cortisol — The Hunger That Comes From Stress

Cortisol may be the most important appetite driver of all, because it is the most misidentified.

When cortisol rises — in response to stress, conflict, poor sleep, overwork, or any perceived threat — it raises blood sugar by prompting the liver to release stored glucose. The blood sugar spike triggers an insulin response. The insulin response drives a blood sugar drop. And the drop is interpreted by the brain as hunger.

This is why stress makes you hungry. Not metaphorically — physiologically. The stress hormone directly creates the metabolic conditions that the brain interprets as a need for food. And the food the stressed brain reaches for is not a salad. It is the fastest available glucose — refined carbohydrates, sugary foods, anything that promises rapid relief from the drop.

The stressed eating that follows is not emotional weakness. It is a cortisol- driven glucose event masquerading as hunger. And because it is driven by a hormone rather than actual caloric need, eating temporarily relieves it — which reinforces the behavior — but does not resolve the underlying stress that created it. Managing cortisol is therefore not separate from managing appetite. It is managing appetite. Everything that calms the nervous system — sleep, movement, community, the morning and evening anchors we will build in Chapter Seven — is an appetite intervention.

Let me tell you about the patients who struggle most with appetite — and when they struggle.

For many of my patients, the hardest moments come at the end of the day — when the obligations are done, the house is quiet, and for the first time since morning there is nothing to do but sit with themselves. The structure that held the day together has fallen away. And that is when the pull toward food arrives.

When I ask what is happening in the evening, the answers are remarkably consistent. The day is done. The obligations are met. The dishes are washed, the kitchen is clean, the family has gone to bed. And for the first time all day, there is nothing to do and no one to serve. This is their time. Their reward for having given everything to everyone else since morning. And the reward is food.

I have a patient — a retired gentleman who spent decades working — who stays up late watching old Westerns. television shows he has watched for years Shows he loved as a young man. And while he watches, he eats. Not out of hunger. Out of the particular comfort that comes from being alone, quiet, unhurried, with no one needing anything from him. The food is part of the ritual of being off-duty. It is what freedom tastes like.

I have a caretaker who spends his days tending to a wife who is seriously ill and adult children with special needs. He loves his family. He has given his life to their care. But by ten o'clock at night, when everyone is settled and the house is quiet, he finally has a moment that belongs only to him. And he fills it with food. Not because he is hungry. Because it is the one uncomplicated pleasure available to him in a day that has been complicated from beginning to end.

One patient put it to me in a way I have never forgotten — the same words I shared in the chapter on the H.E.A.T. model, because they belong here too. Food, she told me, is always available. It never says it's too busy. It never cries at her. It is a constant, willing companion — and in a life where the people she needed were not always there, that constancy became the whole point.

She was not describing gluttony. She was describing loneliness. She was describing, with extraordinary precision, why appetite suppression cannot be solved by hormonal interventions alone. Because some of what drives us toward food runs deeper than hormones — into the relational texture of a person's life. The loneliness that sends someone to the kitchen at ten o'clock at night has a cortisol signature. But cortisol is not the cure. Connection is. It is the pull that fills the space where connection used to be. And connection is something no macronutrient can provide.

As I progressed in my own journey, something shifted in my relationship with food that I had not anticipated and could not have predicted.

I stopped thinking about food constantly.

The food noise — the background hum of food-related thoughts that had characterized my life for years — went quiet. I would wake up not thinking about breakfast. I would finish a meal and simply be done. I could feel the difference between real hunger and the conditioned reach, between the body asking for something it needed and the habituated pattern looking for its familiar cue.

As insulin levels normalized, the blood sugar became steadier. As blood sugar became steadier, the false hunger signals became quieter. As the false hunger signals quieted, I discovered something I had not experienced in years — possibly decades:

I could eat a meal and simply be finished.

Not fighting a craving for something more. Not planning the next eating event before this one was over. Not reaching for something to extend the sensory experience. Just — finished. Satisfied. Done.

That is what a recalibrated appetite feels like. And it is available to you. Not through willpower. Through the restoration of the hormonal system that makes appetite manageable. The pillar does not eliminate hunger. It restores its honesty. It makes hunger a reliable signal again rather than a chronic state.

Here is what suppressing appetite actually looks like in practice.

Protein is the most powerful food-based appetite suppression tool available. It has the highest thermic effect of any macronutrient, meaning the body expends more energy digesting it. It stimulates the release of satiety hormones including GLP-1 and peptide YY. It slows gastric emptying, meaning food stays in the stomach longer and the feeling of fullness lasts. And it has minimal impact on blood sugar and insulin compared to refined carbohydrates, meaning it satisfies without triggering the spike-and-crash cycle that drives false hunger. The combination of protein and healthy fat at a meal is the most effective natural appetite suppression available. Eggs with avocado keeps you full for four hours in a way that cereal simply does not. So does a bowl of lentils or edamame with olive oil — the same principle applies regardless of whether your protein comes from animal or plant sources.

Healthy fats work alongside protein. Fat slows digestion, stimulates satiety hormones, and provides sustained energy without the insulin surge. This is why the low-fat movement that dominated dietary advice for decades actually worsened the appetite problems of millions of people — by removing fat, it removed one of the most powerful natural satiety signals the body has.

Fiber is structural, not optional. Soluble fiber — found in vegetables, legumes, and certain whole grains — slows glucose absorption, feeds the gut microbiome, and extends satiety by physically occupying space in the digestive system and triggering stretch receptors that signal fullness to the brain.

Sleep is an appetite intervention. A single night of poor sleep measurably elevates ghrelin and suppresses leptin — creating the hormonal state of hunger even when the body does not need food. Chronic sleep deprivation creates a sustained state of hormonal hunger that no amount of dietary discipline can fully overcome. If you are not getting adequate sleep and wondering why your appetite feels out of control, part of the answer is in the bedroom.

Stress management is an appetite intervention. Cortisol reduction — through movement, rest, connection, and the practices that regulate the nervous system — directly reduces the cortisol-driven glucose events that the brain misreads as hunger. Every walk you take is not just an insulin efficiency tool. It is a cortisol intervention. It is an appetite tool.

And fasting is perhaps the most comprehensive appetite recalibration tool available. Many people who start fasting expect to be overwhelmed by hunger. What they find instead — after the initial adjustment period — is that the hunger becomes cleaner, clearer, and more manageable than it has ever been. The food noise goes quiet. Not as a side effect. As the physiology working.

But there is a dimension of appetite suppression that goes beyond hormones and macronutrients.

We established in Chapter Three that four forces — Habit, Emotion, Access, and Taste — drive the eating that has nothing to do with physical hunger. These forces do not disappear when insulin levels normalize. They are built into the nervous system, into memory, into the emotional architecture of how you have been living. Suppressing appetite in its full sense requires addressing them.

You can fix the hormonal hunger and still find yourself standing in front of the refrigerator at ten o'clock at night not because your body needs fuel but because something else does. The retired gentleman watching Westerns. The caretaker whose only free hour is after midnight. The patient for whom food is the one companion that never says it is busy. Hormonal interventions help these patients. They are not sufficient by themselves.

The tools for that — the real-time behavioral framework for the moments when the H.E.A.T. forces fire and the decision point arrives — are the subject of Chapter Nine. We will get there. But I want to name it here, in this chapter, because appetite suppression is not complete without it. The hormonal work and the behavioral work are not separate tracks. They are two lanes of the same road.

The person who can hold their breath the longest is not the one with the strongest willpower. It is the one who has learned to breathe more efficiently — who has trained their body to need less air for the same amount of effort. That is what the second pillar does for hunger. Not eliminate it. Recalibrate it. Make it manageable, readable, and honest — so that when you feel the pull to eat, you can tell the difference between your body asking for something it needs and a hormonal system that has been misfiring for years.

The first two pillars address the insulin and the hunger that sustain metabolic disease. The third addresses the substance that is actively driving both.

That is where we go next.

CHAPTER SIX

The Third Pillar — Reduce Sugar

"The most dangerous sugar is the sugar you don't know you're eating."

Years ago, when my wife and I were living in Ohio during my residency, we decided we were going to lose some weight.

I decided I would give up a specific item that I want you to understand the relationship I had with.

Ben and Jerry's Cherry Garcia ice cream.

I do not know how to overstate what that ice cream meant to me. There are foods you eat and foods you love, and then there are foods that have a hold on you that does not respond well to reason. Cherry Garcia was that food. If somebody had walked into the room while I was working and quietly placed a pint of Cherry Garcia on my desk, I would not have been able to focus on anything else until that pint was gone.

But I had made the decision. So I stopped.

And here is the part that surprises people. I did not stop for twenty-four hours. I did not stop for a week. I stopped for almost six months. Six months of walking past freezer aisles. Six months of standing in line behind people whose carts had Ben and Jerry's in them. Six months of letting the craving rise and pass without acting on it. I had built up what felt like real momentum. I had begun to think of myself as a person who did not eat that ice cream anymore.

Then one afternoon my wife called me at the office.

She said, on the way home, can you stop at the store and pick something up. It had nothing to do with ice cream. It was a normal errand. I said yes. I went to the store. I picked up what she had asked for. And I started walking toward the cash register.

You know what was at eye level on the way to the cash register.

Buy one, get one free.

I want you to picture this with me, because the moment is important. I had not gone to the store thinking about ice cream. The thought of ice cream was not on the agenda. I was running an errand for my wife. But the store was not running an errand. The store was working. The store had been built, designed, and stocked by people whose entire job was to make sure that a man walking past that freezer at the end of a long day would do exactly what I was about to do.

I picked up a pint.

And then, as I was walking toward the register, I had what I want to describe honestly as a moment of distorted reasoning. I thought to myself: this is poor consumership. The sign says buy one, get one free. If I do not take both, I am wasting money.

So I went back. And I picked up the second pint. The same flavor. Cherry Garcia.

I paid. I walked out to the car. I started driving home.

And about halfway home, I had a different kind of moment. I realized I could not take the ice cream into the house. My wife was at the house, and I had decided I was not eating Ben and Jerry's Cherry Garcia. If I walked through the door with two pints of it, I was not going to be having ice cream that night. I was going to be having a conversation.

So I pulled the car over to the side of the road.

And I sat there. And I ate them.

I want to say one thing about that moment that I have thought about for years. I do not, as a general rule, ride around with a spoon in my car. I do not have a glove compartment with utensils in it. So when I pulled over, I did not have a spoon. I ate two pints of Cherry Garcia ice cream on the side of the road in Ohio with whatever I had.

By the time I was done, both pints were gone.

I want you to think about what just happened.

For six months I had held the line. I had been disciplined. I had built what I believed was a new identity around not eating that ice cream. And in the span of about forty-five minutes between the freezer and the side of the road, every bit of that came apart. Not because my willpower had suddenly weakened. Not because I had stopped caring about my health. Because the environment changed.

The environment was the variable. The willpower was always going to lose to the environment. And the willpower had been losing to environments like that one my entire adult life. I just did not have the language to see it.

This is what the third pillar is about.

Reducing sugar is not, fundamentally, a project of wanting it less. It is a project of encountering it less. The willpower required to refuse a thing that is not in your house, not in your car, not at eye level on your way to the cash register, is essentially zero. The willpower required to refuse a thing that is six feet from where you are sitting, on sale, in a flavor you have loved since residency, is more than any human being can sustainably produce.

The patients I see who succeed long-term at reducing sugar do not have more willpower than the ones who do not. They have different environments. They have houses without the thing in them. They have grocery routes that do not pass the aisle. They have rituals around the thing — not bans, but containers. They have made the encounter rare instead of constant.

Willpower tires. Environment does not.

If you take one thing from this chapter, take that.

I want to tell you about the carrot cake.

I had been fasting. A colleague at the office found out I had a craving for carrot cake — my favorite. She went out and came back with a beautiful Bundt cake, the cream cheese icing drizzled just right across the top. I was fasting. I knew I was fasting. And I did not eat it.

Instead, I put a piece in the office refrigerator.

Then I put another piece in the refrigerator. And another. By the end of the week, I had stored pieces of carrot cake in the office refrigerator every single day. I told myself I would eat them when I broke my fast. But I also knew — if I am being completely honest — that there was no good reason to store that much carrot cake. None. I was not preserving them for a special occasion. I was hoarding them because my brain did not want them to be unavailable.

Here is what was happening during that week. Every day I walked past the refrigerator, dopamine was building the anticipation. Not just a general craving — a specific, increasingly vivid one. By Wednesday I was noticing the little pieces of pineapple in the batter. By Thursday I was thinking about the coconut on top, the raisins, the way the cream cheese icing had that exact balance of sweet and slightly tangy. I had not noticed any of those details when I first looked at the cake Monday morning. Dopamine was creating them. Dopamine was building a story that became more elaborate and more compelling with every day I did not eat the cake.

On Friday, I ate it.

Then I looked at my continuous glucose monitor.

Two hundred and ninety.

I put my Dexcom data on the screen for my community that night. Numbers in the 150s and 160s all week while I was fasting. Then Friday — 290. I had not seen a number like that in a long time. And I want you to understand something: I am an endocrinologist. I teach this material every week to thousands of people. I know exactly what sugar does to blood glucose. I know the mechanisms. And I still ate the carrot cake because dopamine had spent a week building a case that my prefrontal cortex could not ultimately overrule.

That is not a failure of discipline. That is the biology of sugar. And it is the exact biology we are addressing with the third pillar.

Let me explain what happened that week, because it is happening to you too — probably daily — and understanding the mechanism is the first step toward interrupting it.

When you eat sugar, the brain releases dopamine. Dopamine is the reward neurotransmitter — the pleasure hormone, the motivation hormone, the anticipation hormone. It produces the sensation of satisfaction and reward that the brain then wants to repeat. Sugar is one of the most reliable and powerful dopamine triggers available to most people in most moments. This is not an accident. The foods that produce the strongest dopamine responses have been specifically designed to do so — we covered this in the bliss point section of Chapter Three. But the biology of what happens after that first bite matters just as much.

Dopamine is also activated by anticipation. Not just the eating — the imagining of the eating. When the brain predicts that a reward is coming, it begins releasing dopamine before the reward arrives. This is why I was thinking about pineapple and coconut by Wednesday when I had not even noticed those details on Monday. The dopamine was enriching the memory, adding texture and vividness and sensory detail that were not present in the original experience. It was building a story. And the story was more compelling than the reality had been.

This is not unique to me. Every person who has ever found themselves thinking about a specific food with increasing intensity over hours or days — the brain elaborating the imagined experience, adding detail, making the anticipated pleasure feel more urgent — is experiencing the anticipatory dopamine cycle. The food becomes more vivid in the imagination than it was in reality. And once the dopamine reaches a certain level of activation, the decision not to eat it becomes almost impossible to sustain.

Serotonin joins the cycle when the sugar arrives. Serotonin is the mood stabilizer. When sugar is consumed, serotonin levels rise alongside dopamine, which is why sugar temporarily reduces anxiety, calms agitation, and produces a genuine sense of emotional relief. This is not imagined comfort. This is neurochemistry. Sugar works as a real-time mood regulator — in the short term. It quiets the restless brain. It settles the nervous system. It delivers what it promises, briefly.

Then the sugar is absorbed. Rapidly, because highly processed sugar enters the bloodstream quickly. Blood sugar spikes. Insulin surges. Blood sugar drops. Dopamine fades. Serotonin falls. And what follows is a state that people in addiction recovery describe with precise language:

I know this state. Every person with metabolic disease knows this state.

Restless. Irritable. Discontent.

Those three words are used in recovery communities to name the internal warning signs that precede a relapse — the condition that arises when something the brain has come to depend on is no longer present. And they apply to the sugar crash with startling accuracy. You are not quite comfortable. Something feels slightly off. Everything is a little more irritating than it should be. You cannot fully settle. There is a vague dissatisfaction that has no clear object.

And somewhere in that state, dopamine begins playing the recording: you remember what that felt like. You know what would help.

The cycle restarts. Not because you are weak. Because you are human. Because this is exactly what the cycle was designed — by biology, and by a food environment that learned to take advantage of biology — to produce. Understanding the cycle does not end it. But you cannot interrupt something you cannot see. Naming it is the beginning of working with it.

Let me explain why reducing sugar is the third pillar — and why it is inseparable from the first two.

Every gram of added sugar you consume produces a glucose spike. Every glucose spike produces an insulin response. Every insulin response, repeated across the day, across the week, across the years, contributes to the chronic hyperinsulinemia that drives insulin resistance, weight gain, inflammation, and metabolic disease.

We established in Chapter Four that decreasing insulin is the master lever. Reducing sugar is how you decrease insulin through food. The fasting lowers insulin by creating time without food. The quality of what you eat during your eating window determines whether that work is sustained or immediately undone. You can fast for sixteen hours and spike your insulin dramatically in the eight hours you eat if your food is loaded with added sugar. The fast and the food are not independent. They are a system.

We established in Chapter Five that appetite suppression requires recalibrating the hormonal signals that govern hunger. Sugar is the primary disruptor of those signals. It stimulates ghrelin. It creates leptin resistance. It triggers the dopamine cycle that overrides satiety. A person whose diet is high in added sugar is fighting their appetite hormones with one hand tied behind their back, regardless of how carefully they fast or how intentionally they move.

Reducing sugar is not the most dramatic of the three pillars. But it is the one that holds the other two in place. Without it, the work of the first two pillars is constantly being undermined.

Before we talk about where sugar hides, let me clarify what we mean — because the word sugar is used so broadly that it loses precision.

Not all sugar is the same. Not all carbohydrates are metabolically equivalent. And understanding this distinction protects you from two opposite errors: eliminating foods that support your health because they contain natural sugars, and trusting foods that are sabotaging you because they are marketed as natural.

Natural sugars arrive in the body alongside their original packaging. The fructose in a whole apple comes with fiber, water, pectin, and other compounds that slow its absorption and modulate its metabolic impact significantly. The glucose in a sweet potato comes with fiber and resistant starch that further reduce the glucose response. These foods were never the enemy. Whole fruit, eaten in appropriate quantities, is not the primary driver of metabolic disease.

Added sugars are extracted from their natural sources and incorporated into products during processing — sucrose, high-fructose corn syrup, dextrose, maltose, and the dozens of other names that appear on ingredient lists for the same underlying substance. Added sugars arrive without the fiber and structural compounds that moderate absorption in whole food. They enter the bloodstream rapidly, produce large glucose spikes, and trigger the large insulin responses that, sustained over time, create the conditions for metabolic disease.

The critical question is not whether food contains carbohydrates. It is whether those carbohydrates arrive with the natural fiber and structure that slow their absorption, or stripped of both. A glass of orange juice and a whole orange both contain fruit sugar. The fiber in the whole orange changes everything. The juice delivers the sugar of three to four oranges in a single eight-ounce glass, with no fiber and no moderation. This is why I say to patients: eat the orange, don't drink the orange.

And then there is the question of added sugar entirely — sugar that was never in the food to begin with, put there specifically to enhance palatability and create the dopamine response we just described. This is the sugar we are targeting. Not whole fruit. Not whole vegetables. The sugar that was engineered into the food after it left nature.

Let me walk you through where added sugar actually lives in the modern food supply — starting with the three categories that produce the most surprise in my patients.

Seasonings and Spice Blends

This is the one that catches people completely off guard, because it violates every assumption they have about cooking at home. They are not eating fast food. They are not buying packaged meals. They are cooking with real ingredients. And then they reach for the spice blend — the barbecue rub, the Cajun seasoning, the steak seasoning, the taco mix, the lemon pepper, the garlic herb blend — and add it without a second thought.

It never occurs to most people to read the label on a spice jar. But sugar is one of the most common ingredients in commercial spice blends. It enhances flavor, promotes the browning and caramelization that makes food look and smell appealing, and extends shelf life. A tablespoon of a typical barbecue rub can contain three to five grams of added sugar. A single packet of taco seasoning can contain six to eight grams. The seasoning on a rotisserie chicken purchased from the grocery store often lists sugar among its first five ingredients.

The person who is cooking carefully at home, buying whole ingredients, avoiding obvious sweets, and still cannot get their blood sugar under control is sometimes losing the battle in the spice cabinet. The solution is not to stop seasoning food — food that tastes good is food you will actually eat. The solution is to read the label, choose blends made with herbs and individual spices only, or make your own. Single-ingredient spices contain no added sugar. The blend is where it hides.

Diet Foods and Health Foods

This is the category that produces the most frustration in my practice — and the most important revelations — because the patients most affected are the ones who have been trying hardest.

When the low-fat dietary movement took hold in the 1970s and 1980s, food manufacturers faced a genuine problem. Fat carries flavor. Remove the fat and the food tastes flat, chalky, and unsatisfying. Consumers do not buy food they do not enjoy. So the industry found a solution: replace the fat with sugar. A product could be reformulated to be low in fat, marketed as a healthier choice, and made palatable again through the addition of sugar — often more sugar than the original version contained.

The result is a food landscape in which the products most trusted by health- conscious consumers are sometimes among the most problematic for blood sugar. Low-fat yogurt often contains more added sugar per serving than a scoop of vanilla ice cream. Reduced-fat salad dressing frequently compensates for the missing fat with corn syrup or cane sugar. Granola — which carries a powerful health halo from its association with whole grains and natural ingredients — is typically bound together with honey, syrup, or sugar and contains more grams of sugar per serving than many breakfast cereals marketed to children. Protein bars sold in gyms and health food stores regularly contain twenty to thirty grams of added sugar.

The health halo is one of the more effective marketing approaches the food industry has developed. It creates unearned trust. It allows a product to be associated with health, nature, or wellness in the consumer's mind regardless of its actual nutritional profile. And it specifically targets the people who are already trying — the motivated patients who are making an effort, who are reading labels for fat and calories but not yet for sugar, who cannot understand why their blood sugar is not responding to their careful choices.

When I sit down with a patient in this situation and we go through their food diary together, the revelation is almost always in the health foods. The yogurt they have every morning. The granola they add to it. The protein bar they eat after the gym. The smoothie they make because it seems like a healthy breakfast. The salad dressing on the salad they eat virtuously at lunch. Together, these "healthy" choices can easily represent forty to sixty grams of added sugar before dinner.

Toothpaste, Medications, and the Invisible Sources

When I started wearing a continuous glucose monitor consistently, I discovered something that surprised me even as an endocrinologist.

Every morning, within minutes of brushing my teeth, my blood sugar rose. Not dramatically. But reliably and measurably, every single morning — a small but visible uptick on the monitor, happening before I had eaten anything.

Toothpaste contains sweeteners. Most commercial toothpastes contain saccharin, sorbitol, or other sugar alcohols — partly for taste, partly because these compounds create the texture and foam we associate with a clean mouth. The amounts are small. But when you are fasting, when your blood sugar is at its lowest point of the day and your insulin is quiet, even a small input creates a visible response on a continuous monitor.

Once you start looking for sugar with this level of attention, you find it in places that genuinely surprise you every time. Liquid medications — particularly common forms of antibiotics, cough syrups, antacids, and reflux medications — are sweetened for palatability. Chewable vitamins are essentially gummy candy with supplemental nutrients added. Breath mints and cough drops are almost entirely sugar. Many commonly used supplements come in gummy form that requires sugar to hold its shape and palatability.

None of these sources individually represents a major metabolic threat to most people. But they illustrate a principle that matters enormously for anyone trying to understand their own blood sugar: the modern food and pharmaceutical environment has added sugar to virtually every category of consumable product. It is the default ingredient in anything that needs to taste acceptable. And this means that reducing sugar requires a level of intentional investigation that most people have never thought to apply.

Here is how to read a food label for added sugar, because the label is designed to obscure as much as it reveals.

Start with the Nutrition Facts panel. The "Total Sugars" line includes both natural and added sugars — it tells you how much sugar is in the product but not where it came from. The "Added Sugars" line, which is now mandatory on US labels, tells you how much sugar was put into the product beyond what occurs naturally. This is the number that matters for our purposes.

But the ingredient list is where the real story lives. Sugar hides under more than sixty different names. High-fructose corn syrup. Cane sugar. Beet sugar. Brown sugar. Turbinado sugar. Coconut sugar. Agave nectar. Honey. Maple syrup. Molasses. Dextrose. Maltose. Fructose. Sucrose. Glucose. Corn syrup. Rice syrup. Barley malt. Evaporated cane juice. Some of these names sound natural and therefore healthy. They are all added sugar. The body does not distinguish between organic cane sugar and high-fructose corn syrup at the level of the glucose spike. The spike is the spike.

Ingredients are listed in descending order by weight. If any form of sugar appears in the first three or four ingredients, the product contains a significant amount. But manufacturers have learned to distribute sugar across multiple forms — listing cane sugar, then brown rice syrup, then dextrose, then molasses — so that no single form appears near the top of the list, even though the combined sugar content is substantial. When you see multiple forms of sugar distributed through an ingredient list, that distribution is usually intentional.

Now let me answer the question I hear most often about this pillar.

"Does reducing sugar mean I can never eat anything sweet again?"

No. It means something more nuanced and more sustainable than that.

It means understanding the difference between an occasional intentional choice and a daily default. The carrot cake at a birthday celebration is not what drove the epidemic of type 2 diabetes. The carrot cake logic applied to every weekday, in the form of flavored yogurt and sweetened granola and protein bars and salad dressing, is what drove it. Occasional and intentional is not the same as constant and unconscious. This framework is not about perfection. It is about awareness.

It means learning that the palate is trainable. The taste for sweetness is not a fixed biological constant. It is calibrated by what you expose it to, and it recalibrates faster than most people expect. People who reduce their added sugar intake consistently for thirty to sixty days regularly report that foods they previously found acceptably sweet now taste overwhelmingly so — almost unpleasantly. And foods they previously found bland begin to reveal complexity and flavor they had never tasted. A strawberry starts to taste like something worth paying attention to. A walnut becomes rich in a way it never was before. The palate wakes up when it is no longer being overwhelmed.

It means becoming a label reader — not obsessively or permanently, but initially with enough diligence to build an accurate mental map of where the sugar is in your diet. Most people who do this exercise are shocked. Not by the obvious sources they already knew about. By the accumulation of the sources they had never considered. Once you see the full picture, you cannot unsee it. And once you cannot unsee it, the choices become clearer.

I want to close this chapter with something practical and honest, because I think it is the most useful thing I can say about the third pillar.

When patients walk into my office, they almost always tell me they know what to do. Stop the juice. Stop the soda. Cut the refined carbs. Reduce the processed food. Avoid added sugar. They can name every category that is working against them. They have heard the advice. They know the recommendations. And they look at me and say: so why can I not do it?

The answer is not discipline. The answer is structure.

Think about automatic savings. If you have to manually transfer money from your checking account to your savings account every month, it often does not happen. Not because you do not want to save. Not because you do not know that saving is important. But because the decision requires a deliberate act in a moment when other things are competing for your attention. You forget. You need it for something else. You tell yourself you will do it next month.

But if the transfer is automatic — if it happens the moment your paycheck arrives before you ever see the money — savings happen reliably. Not because you became more disciplined. Because the structure removed the decision from the moment of temptation. You never have to choose between saving and spending because the saving is already done.

Reducing sugar works the same way. The goal is not to be a person who resists sugar every time it appears. That requires willpower applied at the moment of maximum vulnerability — when dopamine is building anticipation, when cortisol has lowered your resistance, when the food is right there in front of you and a week of accumulated craving has made it feel urgent. Willpower at that moment is the least reliable tool available.

The goal instead is to build a structure — in your home, your work environment, your shopping habits, your daily routine — where the decision has already been made. Where the high-sugar foods are not present in the moment of weakness. Where the alternatives are accessible and prepared. Where the environment does the work that willpower was never built to sustain.

I still eat carrot cake. Occasionally, intentionally, with full awareness of what it will do to my blood sugar and acceptance of that as a choice I am making. What I do not do anymore is store carrot cake in the office refrigerator for a week and let dopamine spend seven days building an argument I cannot win. The framework did not make me stop wanting carrot cake. It changed the conditions under which I encounter it. That is the difference between structure and willpower. Structure wins. Willpower tires.

The three pillars are not three separate interventions. They are three angles on the same underlying problem — and when all three are working together, something becomes possible that years of dieting and willpower and medication adjustment never produced.

A metabolism that works with you instead of against you. Blood sugar that reflects what you ate rather than what your hormones have been doing for the past decade. A body that is not broken — because it never was — but that is finally operating in the conditions it was designed for.

That is what the framework delivers. And now it is time to show you how all three pillars come together in a life you can actually live — not a perfect life, not a life without carrot cake, but a structured and intentional life that holds your health even when the days get complicated.

CHAPTER SEVEN

The Pillars in Practice — Building Your Personal Framework

"Consistency does not mean same."

That is the most important thing I can tell you about making the three pillars work in a real life.

Not the science. Not the protocols. Not the optimal fasting window or the ideal macronutrient ratio or the perfect weekly movement target. Those things matter, and we have covered them. But the single insight that separates the people who reverse their diabetes from the people who try and stop trying is this:

Consistency does not mean same.

It means showing up. Every day, in whatever form showing up is possible that day. It means the five-minute walk on the day everything fell apart counts. It means the default meal — the one that is not exciting, not optimal, not what you would choose if you had all the time and all the ingredients in the world — counts. It means the morning that begins with two minutes of stillness instead of thirty still begins with intention.

The people who succeed are not the ones who follow the framework perfectly. They are the ones who never fully stop following it. Who have internalized the difference between a bad day and quitting. Who have built a structure flexible enough to absorb real life and still move forward.

This chapter is about how to build that structure. Not in theory. In the actual conditions of the actual life you are living. Every tool that follows answers the same question: what does showing up actually look like when the day does not go as planned, when the schedule is full, when everything around you is in motion?

Before we talk about what this approach looks like in practice, I want to give you the organizing principle that holds everything together.

Three words. Rhythm. Alignment. Structure.

These are not motivational concepts. They are operational ones. They describe the architecture of a life that moves in a consistent direction even when the details change from day to day.

Rhythm is the general direction of your life — what you say you want, what you are building toward, the identity you are constructing through your daily choices. When I say I want to reverse my diabetes, when I say I want to be metabolically healthy, when I say I want to have energy and clarity and a body that works with me instead of against me — that is my rhythm. It is the direction I have declared. It is the answer to the question: what is this life about?

Alignment is the honest question that follows: are the things I am actually doing taking me in that direction? Not the things I intend to do. The things I do. If my rhythm is metabolic health but I am eating added sugar at every meal, my behavior is not aligned with my rhythm. If I say I want to fast but I am scheduling dinner at a time that makes fasting structurally impossible, I am not aligned. Alignment is not judgment. It is navigation. It is the GPS asking: is this route taking you where you said you want to go? If not, recalculate. Not with guilt. With information.

Structure is what makes alignment sustainable. It is the calendar appointment, the accountability partner, the community you show up to, the default meal in the refrigerator, the morning routine that starts the day before the day has a chance to derail it. Motivation is powerful and unreliable. Structure is less exciting and completely dependable. Motivation gets you started. Structure keeps you going when motivation is nowhere to be found.

When you structure your eating within a consistent window — beginning and closing each day with intention — you are not only building behavioral structure. You are restoring the circadian architecture of hunger regulation that type 2 diabetes disrupts. The disease scrambles the timing signals that govern when hunger rises and falls. Structure repairs them.

Let me give you a real example of what misalignment looks like — and how structure fixes it.

Fasting is one of the most powerful tools in this framework. But I have watched many patients abandon it not because fasting did not work but because they tried to implement it in a way that created unnecessary friction with their actual life.

Here is the scenario I see repeatedly. Someone decides to start fasting. They choose a window — say, they will stop eating at five o'clock in the afternoon. That is their fast. But their family sits down to dinner at six. Which means they are at the table while everyone else is eating, not eating, explaining themselves, fielding questions, managing the social discomfort of being the person doing something different. Eventually they face a choice that should never have been framed as a choice: community or fasting.

Most people choose community. They should. Connection and family cohesion are not obstacles to health. They are components of it. The problem is not that they chose community. The problem is that they designed their fasting window in a way that forced that choice in the first place.

The solution is alignment. Move the eating window to include the family dinner. Eat with your family at six. Close your eating window at seven or seven-thirty. Open it later the next morning. The fasting window is preserved, the family dinner is preserved, and the false tension disappears.

The framework bends to fit the life. The life does not have to break to fit the framework.

This principle applies everywhere. The framework is a tool, not a prison. Its job is to serve your health, which exists inside a real life with real relationships and real obligations. When the framework creates unnecessary friction with the life, the friction is the problem — not the life. Adjust the framework. Maintain the direction.

This brings me to the concept that makes the difference between people who sustain the framework and people who abandon it — and one that most people never arrive at without a structure to guide them.

The non-negotiable minimum.

Not the optimal. Not the ideal. The minimum that happens no matter what. The floor, not the ceiling.

I want to tell you about a patient who understood this better than almost anyone I have worked with. She had been through the cycle many times before she came to me — motivated starts, ambitious plans, early success, then a disruption, then a collapse, then starting over from zero. She was intelligent and she was determined and she kept running into the same wall: when life got hard, the plan required too much, and the whole thing came down at once.

When we worked together, we stopped building the plan from the top down. We built it from the bottom up. I asked her one question: what is the absolute minimum you could do, on the worst possible day you can imagine, that you would still call a win?

She thought about it seriously. She said: a ten-minute walk. I can always do a ten-minute walk. Even if everything else falls apart, I can do that.

That became her floor. On the hard days, ten minutes. On the good days, much more. But never below ten minutes. Never a zero.

There is something else the after-meal walk is doing that I want to name directly, because it matters more for the person with type 2 diabetes than for anyone else. The walk is not only a daily metabolic intervention. It is practice for the hardest moment. Research confirms that a single bout of movement restores postprandial fullness in patients with type 2 diabetes even when the hormonal hunger signals are not cooperating. When polyphagia fires — when the disease is generating a hunger signal that will not soften on its own — movement is the response that works at the biological level, not the behavioral one. But it only works as a crisis response if it is already automatic. A habit you have never built is not available to you in a moment of physiological distress. Every walk you take now, at a time when taking it is relatively easy, is loading that response into your body's memory. You are not just improving your blood sugar today. You are preparing your body to know what to do on the day when your brain may not be able to lead.

Within a few months, something had shifted. The ten-minute floor had not become a ceiling — her good days were still good. But the floor had protected her. The disruptions that had previously collapsed her entire structure now only disrupted the easy parts. The non-negotiable minimum held. And because it held, she never had to start over from zero again. She was always in the game.

Here is how I guide patients through identifying their non-negotiable minimums. Three questions.

What is your one non-negotiable movement? Not your workout goal — your floor. The thing you will do on the worst day, the travel day, the day everything went sideways. For many of my patients this is a ten-minute walk. Some choose five minutes of movement around the house. The specific activity matters less than the commitment: this happens regardless. No day is a zero.

What is your one non-negotiable food choice? Not a meal plan — a default. The meal you can always make, the option that is always available, the choice that requires no decision-making energy because it is already decided. For many people this is eggs and vegetables. For others it is a specific protein and a salad. The default meal is not about perfection. It is about having something solid to reach for when you have no bandwidth for decisions. When everything is uncertain, the default is certain.

What is your one non-negotiable mental anchor? The practice that starts or ends your day with intention. For some this is five minutes of prayer or stillness in the morning. For others it is a brief evening review — not a judgment, an assessment. What did I do today that moved me toward my rhythm? What would I do differently tomorrow? This practice costs almost nothing in time and returns an enormous amount in clarity and direction.

These three non-negotiables are your floor. They are what consistency looks like on the hard days. And the hard days are the ones that determine whether this becomes permanent or temporary. The easy days take care of themselves. Protect the floor, and the floor will protect you.

The non-negotiable minimum gives you the floor for movement and mental anchoring. But the question of what showing up looks like at the table — in a restaurant, at a client dinner, at the family gathering where nothing on offer matches your plan — that question has its own answer.

It is called Balance Bites.

Balance Bites is not a diet. It is not a meal plan with prescribed servings and specific foods at specific times. It is a framework for thinking about food so that every eating decision, wherever you are and whatever options are in front of you, can be made in alignment with your metabolic health.

The seven guiding principles are simple enough to hold in your mind at any table, in any restaurant, at any family gathering.

Whole foods first. Whatever is in front of you, reach for the thing closest to its original form before anything else. The grilled chicken before the breaded one. The roasted vegetables before the casserole. The whole fruit before the juice.

Minimize processing. If the ingredient list is long and full of things you cannot pronounce, that food should not be the center of your plate. This is not a rule that requires reading every label at every meal. It is a direction that guides the default choices.

No added sugar as the target. Not the absolute rule that triggers guilt when it is broken, but the direction you are always moving toward. The birthday cake at the celebration is a choice you make with awareness. The added sugar in the salad dressing and the spice blend and the protein bar is the unconscious accumulation that does the real damage.

Protein and healthy fat at every meal. These are your satiety tools, your hormone stabilizers, your metabolic foundation. They are not optional extras for people who have time and resources. They are the non-negotiable center of the plate.

Starchy and non-starchy vegetables understood and chosen deliberately. Not eliminated — chosen. Knowing that a third of a cup of rice will produce a different glucose response than a cup of broccoli allows you to make an informed decision rather than an accidental one.

Portion awareness. Not calorie counting. Awareness. Eating slowly, stopping at satisfaction rather than fullness, recognizing that the satiety signal takes twenty minutes to reach the brain after the stomach has received enough. The person who eats slowly discovers they need less food to feel satisfied than they thought.

Tasty and enjoyable. This one is non-negotiable for a different reason. Sustainable means it fits the person you are becoming — not the person who white-knuckles every meal, but the person who has redesigned their relationship with food so that what serves their health is also what feels normal, natural, and genuinely satisfying. That does not happen overnight. The palate adapts. What feels unfamiliar at the start soon feels familiar. Season your food. Explore preparation. Give yourself permission to keep discovering what works. The goal is not perfection at the table. It is a way of eating you have made yours.

Let me tell you how one patient applied Balance Bites in a situation that seemed impossible.

He was a traveling salesman. On the road four days a week, eating every meal in a different city, at client dinners, airport terminals, hotel restaurants. He told me when we started that he could not do this framework because his life did not allow it. Every meal was a negotiation he did not control.

We spent one session going through Balance Bites together and applying it to his actual travel reality. At the airport: eggs or grilled protein at any sit-down restaurant — or edamame for a plant-based option — water instead of juice, nuts instead of the packaged snacks at the gate. At client dinners: protein and vegetables as the base of the plate, skip the bread basket, order sauces on the side. At the hotel: request a room refrigerator, keep hard-boiled eggs or deli turkey for the morning, avoid the continental breakfast which is almost entirely refined carbohydrates and added sugar.

He came back three months later having lost twenty-two pounds. His A1C had dropped by two points. He had not followed the framework perfectly — there were client dinners where he ate things that were off the plan, and there were days on the road where the only available option was genuinely limited. But he had internalized the direction. He was no longer making accidental choices. He was making intentional ones inside imperfect circumstances. That is what Balance Bites is designed to produce.

Balance Bites handles the food side of the question. But movement has its own version of the same problem: the day when the gym is not available, the walk did not happen, and the only thing standing between you and a zero is the willingness to do something small.

For that day, there is one answer.

The five-minute plan.

Not the full workout. Not the ideal meal. The five-minute version of everything that matters. The five-minute walk they can take anywhere — around the terminal, around the hotel block, around the parking lot. The default meal that exists at almost every airport and hotel — eggs, a salad, grilled protein. The five-minute morning anchor that starts the day with intention regardless of the time zone or the meeting schedule or how late the flight arrived the night before.

The five-minute plan exists because the most dangerous moment in any health journey is not the hard day. It is the day you tell yourself you cannot do anything because you cannot do everything. The all-or-nothing trap. The zero day that becomes two zero days that becomes a week that becomes the quiet end of the attempt, with no dramatic moment of quitting but just a gradual drift back to the default.

Five minutes breaks that pattern. Five minutes says: I showed up. I am still in this. Today was not a zero. Tomorrow we build from here.

I have had patients tell me that the five-minute plan felt silly at first — that five minutes did not feel like enough to matter. What they discovered is that the value of the five-minute plan is not the five minutes themselves. It is the identity it protects. The person who does the five-minute walk on the travel day is still a person who moves. The person who skips movement entirely for four days of a business trip has started a different story. The five minutes is not the point. Staying in the story is the point.

The structure that my most successful patients share is not complicated. It has two bookends and a direction.

The morning bookend starts the day before the day takes over. It does not have to be long — fifteen minutes is enough. But it needs to exist and it needs to be non-negotiable. Stillness. Prayer. A brief review of intentions. The walk that happens before the phone is checked and the demands begin. Whatever form it takes, the morning bookend is a declaration: I am the author of this day, not the recipient of it.

The evening bookend closes the loop. It is brief — five to ten minutes — and it asks three questions: What did I do today that moved me toward my rhythm? What happened that did not? What is one thing I will do differently tomorrow? This is not self-criticism. It is calibration. It is the difference between drifting through your life and designing it.

Between those two bookends is a day. It will not always go as planned. The meeting will run long. The travel will disrupt the routine. The family will need something that was not on the schedule. The food options will not be ideal. That is not a failure of the design. That is life inside the design. This approach is not built for ideal conditions. It is built to function in actual ones.

Let me show you what a real day inside this framework looks like — not the optimal version. The sustainable one.

The morning bookend happens before anything else. Fifteen minutes of stillness or prayer or quiet intention, then movement

— a walk, even a short one. Not because it is the most efficient exercise protocol in existence. Because it sets insulin sensitivity, regulates cortisol, and signals to the brain that today is a day when the body is being cared for. The walk is a vote for the identity.

The eating window opens at a time aligned with the family schedule and the fasting goal. The first meal is built around protein and healthy fat — something that opens the eating window without generating an insulin surge. That might be eggs with vegetables, or a plant-based option like tofu, tempeh, or legumes prepared with olive oil. No refined carbohydrates, no added sugar. Not because these are forbidden. Because this meal keeps blood sugar stable and appetite quiet for hours, which makes every subsequent decision in the day easier. Starting right creates metabolic momentum.

During the day, when the coworker's candy bowl appears, when the meeting has pastries, when the afternoon craving arrives right on schedule — the C.O.P.E. framework is available. Clarify what is actually happening.

Observe where it lives in the body. Pause long enough to interrupt the automatic reach. Execute the aligned choice. This is not a lengthy process. It takes thirty seconds. But those thirty seconds are the difference between a designed moment and a default one.

The afternoon may bring a meal or a snack, depending on the eating window. If eating, it follows Balance Bites principles — directionally. The question is always: is this moving me toward my rhythm or away from it? Not: is this perfect? Directional is good enough. Directional, maintained consistently, produces transformation.

The eating window closes at a time that preserves the fasting window without creating family friction. The evening meal — if it falls within the window — is eaten at the table, slowly, with presence. The body's satiety signals are given time to register. The meal ends when there is satisfaction, not when there is fullness.

The evening bookend closes the day. Five minutes. Three questions. Calibration, not judgment. And then sleep — protected, prioritized, treated as the metabolic intervention it actually is. The phone is not in the bedroom. The room is dark. The conditions for quality sleep are not left to chance, because quality sleep is not a luxury. It is a metabolic necessity.

Here is what happens when this structure is maintained consistently — over weeks and months.

The insulin levels begin to normalize. The appetite recalibrates. The food noise that has been running in the background for years begins to quiet. The weight begins to shift. The A1C begins to move. The medications begin to be reviewed and reduced. The energy that was being consumed by fighting the biology becomes available for living.

And something else happens that is harder to quantify but no less real. The identity shifts.

You stop being a person who is trying to manage a chronic disease and start being a person who is building a life by design. The framework stops feeling like something you are following and starts feeling like something you are. The walk is no longer a task on a list. It is what you do. The food choices are no longer negotiations you have to win. They are expressions of who you have become.

That shift — from compliance to identity — is what makes it permanent. Diets end. Identities do not.

I have watched patients reach that shift. It does not happen at a dramatic moment. It happens quietly — when they realize they have not thought about quitting. When the framework is no longer something they are doing but something they are. That is when you know the work is finished in the most important sense: not because the blood sugar is in range, but because the person who produced that blood sugar has changed.

The three pillars give you the metabolic foundation. Rhythm, Alignment, and Structure give you the daily architecture. Balance Bites gives you the food philosophy. The non-negotiable minimums give you the floor that prevents the zero days. The morning and evening bookends give you the container that holds it all.

But there is a dimension of this journey that no operational framework fully addresses on its own. Because the conditions that created metabolic disease were not just dietary and behavioral. They were emotional. They were shaped by stress, by the relationship between feeling and eating, by patterns of response to difficulty that the H.E.A.T. model names but does not by itself resolve.

Part Three of this book is about those invisible forces — the ones that operate underneath the clinical framework and determine whether the framework holds when life gets genuinely hard. The ones that fired when the divorce proceedings started and the blood sugar normalized overnight once they ended. The ones that sent blood sugar spiking before a stressful person even walked through the door. The ones that registered a recurring anxiety on a glucose monitor as reliably as a clock. These are the forces that no pillar alone can address — and understanding them changes everything about how you approach the work ahead.

Understanding those forces — and having real tools for navigating them in real time — is what separates the approach that works for a few months from the one that works for a lifetime.

We begin with the brain.

PART THREE

The Invisible Forces

CHAPTER EIGHT

The Emotional Brain and Your Metabolism

"The struggle with diabetes often has nothing to do with the disease. It has everything to do with the life around it."

Whenever I give a presentation about metabolism and diabetes, there is an exercise I sometimes do.

I ask for a volunteer. Someone comes up to the front. I introduce myself. I ask their name. I ask how long they think they can hold their breath. Most people, off the top of their head, will say something like twenty or thirty seconds. They are usually a little embarrassed by the number, like they think they should be able to do better.

Then I reach into my wallet. And I pull out twenty dollars.

I tell the volunteer the twenty dollars is theirs if they can hold their breath for two minutes.

People laugh, because two minutes sounds absurd compared to the twenty seconds they just estimated. But I want you to understand the math of the offer. I am asking the volunteer to hold their breath for six times as long as they think they can. And I am paying real money to do it. Not a participation prize. Not a token. Twenty dollars in their pocket, in front of a room of people, for doing something the body is fully capable of doing in theory.

I tell the volunteer to take some big deep breaths. I tell them not to cheat — not to breathe shallow, not to gasp at the start. I get a timekeeper from the audience. I count them in.

They hold their breath.

Five seconds. Ten. Fifteen. Twenty.

Around twenty, the face starts to change. The shoulders rise. The eyes widen slightly. The volunteer is doing the math everybody does at this point in the exercise, calculating how much further they can push.

Twenty-five. Thirty.

Thirty-five seconds.

They break.

They gasp. They bend forward. The room applauds. They stand up, embarrassed and laughing at the same time. I shake their hand and I thank them and I ask them to stay at the front for one more minute, because the point of the exercise has not landed yet.

I turn to the audience and I ask the question.

I ask: did they want the twenty dollars?

Of course they wanted the twenty dollars. They were a volunteer in front of a room. Everyone wants the twenty dollars.

I ask: were they motivated?

Of course they were motivated. They were holding their breath for as long as they could.

I ask: did they believe they could do it?

They thought they had a chance. Otherwise they would not have tried.

I ask: then why did they stop?

There is usually a pause in the room when I ask that question, because people know the answer but they have to find the words for it. And the answer, when it comes, is the entire point of the exercise.

They stopped because the body made them stop.

It did not consult their will. It did not check with their goals. It did not weigh the twenty dollars against the desire to follow through. The body had a chemistry running underneath the surface that the conscious mind had no vote in. As they held their breath, carbon dioxide built up in the blood. Receptors in the brainstem registered the rise and triggered an alarm. The alarm did not ask permission. It did not negotiate. It simply overrode every conscious commitment they had made about not breathing for two minutes, because the body had decided the situation was no longer survivable on those terms.

The body made them do what it wanted them to do.

Now I want you to sit with that, because it is the most important thing in this chapter.

Most of what we call emotional eating is exactly the same phenomenon as the volunteer at thirty-five seconds.

You have decided you are not going to eat the thing. You have committed to it. You have prepared for it. You believe in your goals. You are motivated. And then somewhere around the equivalent of thirty-five seconds — after a hard day, after an argument, after a moment of grief or stress or loneliness — your body takes over. The hand reaches into the cabinet. The car turns into the drive-through. The ice cream is in front of you and you do not remember exactly how you got there.

What you are experiencing in those moments is not weakness. It is chemistry.

There are drivers underneath the surface that have been deciding things long before your conscious mind got the chance to weigh in. Cortisol, the stress hormone, rises during a hard day and signals the brain to seek high-density calories — not because you are emotionally fragile, but because your body is doing what it was designed to do when it perceives a threat. Ghrelin, the hunger hormone, rises after poor sleep and floods the system with a demand that no amount of willpower can fully silence. Insulin swings can drop your blood sugar to a level where the brain registers a survival emergency, and at that point the brain does not care about your weight goals, your A1C, or the promise you made to yourself this morning. It cares about glucose. Now.

These are the equivalent of carbon dioxide building up in the blood of a person holding their breath. They are not negotiable. They are not a referendum on your character. They are the body asserting itself with the same authority it asserts when it makes you breathe.

The trap most patients fall into is to interpret this as moral failure. They tried, they believed, they wanted, and they ate the thing anyway. So something must be wrong with them.

Something must be missing. Other people manage. Why can they not.

Here is what is wrong. They are trying to win the equivalent of a two-minute breath-hold by trying harder.

It does not work that way. Trying harder is not the variable.

Reducing the demand — meeting the underlying chemistry so that the body does not have to assert itself — is the variable. If the volunteer had not been holding their breath, no amount of motivation would have been required. The breath would have come naturally, on its own, without crisis. The conscious mind would not have had to fight anything.

That is what the rest of this book is about.

—

I want to say something to the person reading this who has been carrying the weight of this for years.

Maybe you have been telling yourself, for as long as you can remember, that you are weak. That something is broken in you. That other people can do this and you cannot, and the difference is character, and you have come up short. Maybe you have lain awake at night wondering what is wrong with you that you cannot stop doing the thing you keep promising yourself you will stop doing.

If that is you, I want you to hear me carefully.

It was not weakness. It was never weakness.

It was a body with unmet needs doing what bodies do when their needs go unmet for long enough.

You have been losing a fight you were never going to win on those terms — not because you are not strong, but because the fight itself was the wrong fight. You cannot out-discipline biology. Nobody can. The shame you have been carrying for not being able to do something nobody can do is a weight you have been wearing for nothing.

You can put it down.

The body is not your enemy. It has been trying to tell you something the whole time. The day you stop fighting it is the day the fight ends.

That day is closer than you think.

I want to tell you about a pattern I have seen hundreds of times in twenty years of clinical practice.

A patient comes in for a follow-up. Their food has been consistent. Their fasting has been consistent. Their movement has been consistent. By every measure of the framework we have built together, they have been doing the work. And yet their blood sugar numbers have not moved the way they should. Sometimes they have gotten worse.

I ask about the food. Nothing unusual. I ask about the fasting. On track. I ask about movement. Yes. And then — because I have learned to ask — I ask about the life.

And that is where the real answer lives.

Let me give you three examples from my own practice that illustrate this more clearly than any explanation I could offer.

The first is a woman whose blood sugars we had been struggling to control for some time. We adjusted her medications. We evaluated her food log. We looked at her activity, her sleep, every clinical variable we could measure. Nothing explained the numbers. Finally I sat down with her and said: I want to understand what is happening in your life right now — not just the numbers, but what you are carrying. Walk me through your days.

She told me she was going through a divorce.

We had been adjusting her medications for months. And the actual driver of her blood sugar — the chronic cortisol load of a marriage ending, of legal proceedings, of a life being divided and restructured — had never entered the clinical conversation because nobody had thought to ask.

Once the divorce was finalized, her blood sugar came down into the normal range. Almost overnight. Not because she changed anything she was eating. Because the cortisol load she had been carrying finally lifted.

The second example stays with me for its precision.

I had a patient with a continuous glucose monitor, and as we reviewed her data together we noticed a consistent pattern: her blood sugar spiked every morning around six-thirty. We went through everything. Her food the night before. Her sleep. Her morning routine. Nothing explained that specific window.

So I asked her: what happens at six-thirty in the morning?

She thought about it and said: nothing happens at six-thirty. But at seven o'clock, John comes to work.

John was her coworker. They did not get along. And every morning, before John had even arrived, her nervous system had already begun preparing for his presence. The anticipatory stress — the cortisol that rose in response to what was coming rather than what had already happened — was releasing glucose into her bloodstream at six-thirty every morning with the reliability of an alarm clock.

She was not eating anything at six-thirty. John was not even there yet. But her blood sugar did not care. It was responding to the cortisol. And the cortisol was responding to John.

The third example involves a young patient — a high school student, an A student.

When we looked at her glucose monitor data, her blood sugars were excellent in the morning, excellent in the evening. But right around ten o'clock every school day morning, her blood sugar began to spike.

We looked at her schedule. At ten o'clock, she had math.

She was not failing math. She was getting good grades. But math was the class that stressed her. And that ordinary, consistent low-level anxiety, repeated every school day at ten o'clock, was generating enough cortisol to produce a measurable, consistent glucose spike.

Her numbers were fine the rest of the day. Math class was not a food event. It was a cortisol event.

But the story that has stayed with me longest from all these years of clinical practice — the one I tell most often because it captures something the others do not — involves a fourth patient.

Her husband found her standing fully clothed in a running shower, eating a Snickers bar so he would not see her. I will tell you the full story in Chapter Eleven, where it belongs. But here is what it told me about shame:

That is not a willpower failure. That is what shame does to a person over decades of living with a disease in a culture that treats the disease as a moral verdict. She was not hiding the Snickers bar. She was hiding from the judgment about herself that she had come to expect from the people who loved her most.

And I understood her completely. Because I had been hiding for twenty-five years. Not in a shower — but in clinic rooms, in professional language, in the gap between what I was teaching and what I was living. The shame of her story was not foreign to me. It was familiar.

What we hide does not go away. It just eats in private.

The emotional brain is not separate from the metabolic problem. It is often the metabolic problem's primary driver. Shame raises cortisol. Cortisol raises blood sugar. And the hiding that shame produces — from family, from physicians, from the community that might have helped — removes the very support that might have changed the conditions.

These four patients — the woman going through a divorce, the woman whose coworker arrived at seven, the student who had math at ten, and the woman in the shower — illustrate something I want every person reading this book to understand completely:

Your blood sugar is not only responding to what you eat. It is responding to your life.

Here is what is happening inside the body in each of those situations.

Chronic stress activates the hypothalamic-pituitary-adrenal axis — the HPA axis, the body's primary stress response system. The hypothalamus signals the pituitary gland. The pituitary signals the adrenal glands. The adrenal glands release cortisol.

Cortisol is not a villain. It is a survival hormone. Under acute stress — a genuine physical threat, a crisis that demands immediate action — cortisol does exactly what it should. It raises blood sugar by signaling the liver to release stored glucose. It suppresses digestion and reproduction and redirects energy toward the muscles and the brain.

The problem is not cortisol. The problem is what happens when the stress is not acute but chronic — when the emergency never resolves, when the threat is not a predator you can outrun but a divorce, a coworker, a math class, a mortgage, a grief, a shame carried so long it feels like part of who you are.

Under chronic stress, cortisol remains elevated as a sustained background level. And elevated cortisol keeps the liver releasing glucose into the bloodstream even when you have not eaten. The liver does not know the difference between a physical threat and a psychological one. It responds to the cortisol signal the same way either way. Glucose goes up. Insulin goes up in response. And the cycle that drives insulin resistance continues — not because of what you ate for breakfast, but because of what you are carrying.

There is a fourth type of patient I want to describe — one whose story illustrates the domains of health in a way the others do not.

She was intelligent. Informed. She had been diabetic for years and knew the clinical landscape well. Her A1C had climbed into the 14s. Every visit, we had the same conversation. Food. Exercise. Sleep. Medication. She would nod. She would try. Nothing changed.

At some point I had to stop and say: something else is going on. Talking about food is not the answer. Talking about not eating is not the answer. What is the underlying issue that is driving this?

What came out over the next several conversations was not a food problem. It was a life problem. Relational tension that had been building for years. Career dissatisfaction. Financial pressure. A grief she had never fully processed. A loneliness she had never named.

All of it was showing up in her metabolism. Not because these things directly caused diabetes — but because each of them was activating the cortisol response that was raising her glucose independently of anything she ate. And more than that: each of them was activating the H.E.A.T. forces that were driving her eating.

This is one of the most important clinical insights I can offer you:

Metabolic situations often have nothing to do with the disease process. They have everything to do with the domains of life.

Until the life domains are addressed — the relational, the emotional, the vocational, the financial, the spiritual — metabolic improvements tend to be temporary.

I lived this myself.

There was a period several years into building my practice — while simultaneously building Woode Life Design, while being a husband and a father, while managing my own metabolic health, carrying everything that comes with it — when I had quietly normalized a level of stress load that was, by any honest measure, unsustainable.

I was not in crisis. I was functioning. I was producing. But I had been running at what I can only describe as a permanent orange alert for so long that I had stopped noticing it. The background hum of cortisol had become my baseline. The slightly shortened fuse. The reaching for food at ten in the evening. The difficulty being fully present at the dinner table even when I was physically there.

What I did not understand yet was that I was describing a metabolic state, not a character trait. The chronic cortisol was raising my blood sugar independently of my food choices. When I finally understood this — not as a concept but as a personal reality — everything changed. Not because I immediately fixed the stress.

Because I stopped calling it something it wasn't. Overload, unlike personality, can be addressed.

When I say stress management, I do not mean bubble baths and positive thinking.

I mean specific, physiologically grounded practices that reduce cortisol, regulate the nervous system, and create the internal conditions that make metabolic health possible.

Movement as Cortisol Intervention

Every walk you take is a cortisol intervention. Physical activity — particularly moderate aerobic movement like walking — activates the parasympathetic nervous system, which counterbalances the sympathetic activation of the stress response. It lowers circulating cortisol. It clears the glucose that cortisol has released into the bloodstream. The person who walks every morning is not just improving their insulin sensitivity. They are starting the day with a cortisol reset that changes the metabolic context for every subsequent choice.

Sleep as Hormonal Reset

Poor sleep elevates cortisol. Elevated cortisol disrupts sleep. The cycle is self-reinforcing and metabolically devastating. People who consistently get adequate sleep show measurably better insulin sensitivity, lower fasting glucose, healthier cortisol rhythms, and better appetite regulation — regardless of diet. Sleep is not a lifestyle preference. It is a metabolic intervention.

Community as Stress Buffer

Chronic loneliness produces a sustained stress response that elevates cortisol, increases inflammation, and worsens insulin resistance. Community is not a soft add-on to a diabetes management framework. It is a cortisol management strategy. The accountability partner, the support group, the show you show up to every week — these are physiological interventions that reduce the hormonal load that drives blood sugar.

Visualization and the Grounded Mind

One of the practices I use with patients in my exam room is a structured visualization and grounding exercise that produces measurable reductions in stress response over time.

I ask the patient to close their eyes. I walk them through slow, deliberate breathing — the same four-second inhale, two-second hold, four-second exhale pattern we use in the C.O.P.E. framework. As they breathe, I ask them to bring to mind a specific time and place where they felt completely calm. Not a general idea of calm — a specific memory. The sights. The sounds. The smells.

For me, that place is St. Simons Island off the coast of Georgia. I know the feeling of planning that trip — blocking off the days, thinking through the drive down I-65 to I-20 across to the Georgia coast, the moment we cross onto the island. The hotel room with the turned-down bed and the small chocolates on the sheet. When I go there in my mind, I am fully there.

I then anchor them back to the present room — a sound in the environment, the hum of the air conditioning, the ticking of a clock — and count them back slowly. Five. Eyes opening slightly. Four. A little more. Three. Two. One. Fully present.

The instruction I give them is this: you do not have to go anywhere to go there. You can be in a meeting, in traffic, at the end of a hard clinic day — and you can transport yourself to that place for thirty seconds. The cortisol does not know the difference between real and vividly imagined. The parasympathetic response activates either way.

I have a patient who practices this twice a day — at nine in the morning and at three in the afternoon. Two minutes each time. The improvement in her stress levels — and in her blood sugar — over the months she has been doing this has been significant enough that we have reduced her medication.

The Morning and Evening Anchors

The morning anchor — the stillness, the prayer, the intentional beginning before the day's demands arrive — sets the cortisol baseline for the day. The nervous system that enters the day from a regulated state has more capacity available at three in the afternoon than the nervous system that was reactive from the moment the alarm went off.

The evening anchor supports the cortisol decline that healthy sleep requires. The person who is reviewing emails and solving problems at ten o'clock at night is maintaining a cortisol elevation that delays sleep onset and reduces sleep quality. The evening anchor — the five-minute review, the transition ritual, the deliberate closing of the day — is sleep preparation. It is also blood sugar preparation.

There is one more dimension of this chapter that connects the cortisol story back to the H.E.A.T. model.

When cortisol rises, blood sugar rises. When blood sugar rises and then falls, the brain interprets the drop as a need for more glucose. The H.E.A.T. Emotion force fires. The reach toward food begins. And the food that gets reached for is almost never a salad. It is the fastest available glucose — the refined carbohydrate, the sweet thing, the food that promises rapid relief.

The emotional eating is not separate from the metabolic disease. It is one of its mechanisms. Cortisol creates the biological conditions that make emotional eating feel urgent and necessary. This loop — stress, cortisol, glucose, insulin, resistance, more stress — is the hidden engine of type 2 diabetes in millions of people who have been told their problem is what they eat.

Their problem is what they carry.

So what do we do with this?

First, we name it. The emotional and psychological environment is a metabolic environment. If you have been doing everything right and your numbers still will not move, ask yourself honestly: what am I carrying? What is the cortisol load that my labs are reflecting?

Second, we address it with the same seriousness we bring to dietary change. The walks, the sleep, the community, the morning and evening anchors, the visualization practice — these are not lifestyle enhancements. They are cortisol management strategies with direct metabolic consequences.

Third, we build the behavioral tools that interrupt the stress-eat cycle in real time. Because knowing that cortisol drives blood sugar does not, by itself, stop the reach toward the refrigerator when the difficult phone call ends. For that — for the moment between the cortisol surge and the eating behavior — you need a tool that works in real time.

That tool is the subject of the next chapter.

It is called C.O.P.E.

CHAPTER NINE

C.O.P.E. — A Framework for the Moments That Undo You

"The moment between the trigger and the action is where everything is decided."

My son was sick and I needed to get orange juice.

That was the entire mission. Go in, get the juice, come back out. It was late. It had been a long day. No distractions. Just orange juice.

As I walked into the store and turned toward the juice aisle, I passed the bakery. The woman there was tidying up — the store was getting ready to close — and she looked up and said: we just put out some carrot cake.

In that split second, something in my brain said: you've had a long day. You deserve that carrot cake.

I walked over. I looked at it. It looked good. And I grabbed a piece. I was going to feel comfortable. This was going to lower my cortisol. This was going to help me feel a certain way.

As I started walking away, she said: have you tried the pumpkin spice cheesecake? Everybody's been talking about it.

I got some of that too.

And as I was eating it on the way home, I was thinking: why am I eating this? I'm not hungry. But I was in a mood. I came for juice. I left with carrot cake and cheesecake and the juice. And somewhere between the bakery and the car, the decision had already been made without me fully participating in it.

That moment — the drift, the trigger, the automatic reach — is what the C.O.P.E. framework is built to interrupt.

Not to prevent you from ever eating carrot cake. Not to make you a person who never drifts. But to create a moment of awareness between the trigger and the action — long enough for the intentional self to rejoin the conversation.

C.O.P.E. stands for Clarify, Observe, Pause, and Execute. Each step has a specific job. Together they move you from triggered to intentional in a sequence that works with your neurology rather than against it.

Let me explain what is happening in the brain when you drift into the bakery, or reach for the refrigerator after the hard phone call, or find yourself eating something you did not decide to eat.

Your brain operates on two primary systems. The first is fast, automatic, and emotional. It processes information in milliseconds, operates below conscious awareness, and is designed for speed. This system — closely associated with the amygdala — keeps you alive by responding to threat before the thinking brain has time to deliberate.

The second system is slower, deliberate, and rational. The prefrontal cortex — the part of the brain that knows you are trying to reverse your diabetes, that remembers the framework, that can weigh the carrot cake against the goal — operates here.

The problem is sequence. The amygdala fires first. Always. By the time the thinking brain arrives, the hand is already reaching. This is what neuroscientists call an amygdala hijack. It is not a character flaw. It is architecture.

The only way to interrupt this sequence is to create a pause. A deliberate gap between the trigger and the response. Long enough for the prefrontal cortex to come online. Long enough for the designed intention to reassert itself over the automatic default.

I use an analogy when I teach this that I want to share here.

When a heart goes into a dangerous arrhythmia, we use a defibrillator. Most people think the defibrillator starts the heart. It does not. It stops it. The shock interrupts the chaotic electrical activity so completely that the heart goes silent for a moment. And in that silence, the part of the heart that is supposed to be in charge — the sinoatrial node, the natural pacemaker — can reassert its rhythm.

The pause in C.O.P.E. is the defibrillator. It does not start anything. It stops the chaos long enough for the part of you that is supposed to be in charge — your values, your intentions, your designed self — to reassert its rhythm.

C — Clarify

The first step is to identify what is actually happening.

Clarify asks two questions. First: what is the external trigger? What just happened, or is about to happen, that set this in motion? The argument. The deadline. The late night. The loneliness. The visual cue of something in the bakery case. The habit context of the couch after dinner.

Second: what story is your mind telling about that trigger?

Here is something important to understand: the event itself has no power until you give it meaning. Think of it like a shell — an empty form waiting for something to animate it. The moment you interpret the event, you infuse it with life. Your boss's comment, your spouse's tone, your unfinished project — these become threats not because they are threats but because of the story you assign to them. And that story — not the event — is what drives the emotion. And the emotion — not the hunger — is what drives the eating.

Three thought patterns show up most often when the amygdala has taken over. Catastrophizing — turning a difficult moment into total disaster. All- or-none thinking — if the report has one weak section the whole thing is worthless, if I ate one cookie the whole day is ruined. And justifying — convincing yourself that the eating is deserved, or necessary, or not that bad, when you already know the truth.

Clarify does not ask you to change the trigger. It asks you to see it clearly. To separate the event from the meaning you have assigned to it. Because once you can see the distinction, the emotion loses some of its power — and you gain some of yours back.

When I was at the grocery store with the carrot cake, I was not hungry. I was tired and carrying the weight of a long day. The carrot cake had nothing to do with my son's orange juice. It had everything to do with a brain looking for something to make the day feel better. Clarifying means naming that honestly, out loud, even if only to yourself.

O — Observe

The second step is to turn attention inward and read what your body is telling you.

Emotions do not stay in the brain. They show up in the body first. The chest tightens. The jaw clenches. The breathing becomes shallow. The stomach contracts. The shoulders rise. These are not random physical sensations. They are the body's vocabulary for emotional states. And most of us have never been taught to read it.

The five-step Observe sequence works like this:

One — take a deep breath. Not a dramatic breath. One real breath, deep enough to begin activating the parasympathetic nervous system. This initiates the pause at a physiological level. The sympathetic nervous system — the fight-or-flight activation — begins to yield.

Two — scan your body from head to toe. Are you holding tension in your shoulders? Is your jaw clenched? Is your heart rate elevated? Is your stomach churning? You are not judging these sensations. You are noticing them. Observing without verdict.

Three — connect the body symptoms to an emotion. The tightness in the chest is anxiety. The clenched fists are anger. The hollowness in the stomach is loneliness. The restlessness is boredom. The heaviness is grief or exhaustion. The body knows before the mind names it.

Four — name the emotion. Not a vague name. A specific one. Not "I feel bad" but "I feel anxious about the presentation" or "I feel lonely in a way that has been building for days." Research shows that naming an emotion specifically — not a vague label like

"I feel bad" but the precise word for what you are feeling — actually reduces the intensity of the emotional response in the brain. Naming it does not eliminate it. But it reduces its intensity and creates distance between you and the feeling. You shift from being inside the emotion to observing it.

Five — acknowledge the emotion without judgment. This is perhaps the hardest step. We are not comfortable sitting with discomfort. We have spent years learning to buffer it rather than be in it. Acknowledging means saying: this emotion is present. It is valid. It is a temporary state. And I do not have to act on it impulsively right now.

P — Pause

The third step is the defibrillator.

The pause is not a long event. It does not require a quiet room or twenty minutes of reflection. It is a deliberate interruption of the automatic sequence — long enough for the prefrontal cortex to come back online.

Here are three pause techniques that work in real moments:

The breathing protocol: inhale for four seconds, hold for two, exhale for four. Repeat two to three times. This is not complicated. It is biochemistry. The extended exhale activates the vagus nerve, which triggers the parasympathetic response. Heart rate slows. Cortisol begins to decline. The prefrontal cortex gets the window it needs.

The grounding technique: find five things in your environment you can see. Then identify five sounds you can hear. This forces the brain out of the emotional loop and into the present moment. It is not meditation. It is a circuit interrupt. You are holding onto the desk, connecting to something physical, and pulling your awareness back to the room you are actually in rather than the story your brain is running.

The physical step away: remove yourself from the triggering environment if at all possible. Walk to a different room. Step outside for sixty seconds. The physical distance from the trigger reduces the brain's threat response. You cannot fully pause inside the bakery.

One thing I want to be direct about: pausing is not natural. Your amygdala is conditioned, has been conditioned for decades, to respond to triggers without consulting the prefrontal cortex first. The pause does not happen automatically in the moment. It happens automatically only after you have practiced it enough times when you were not in crisis.

This is why I have an alarm on my phone that goes off three times a day. At nine in the morning, at noon, and at mid-afternoon. The alarm says: are you willing right now to do what it takes to be successful? It is not a long pause. It is a few seconds. A breath. A check-in. But those three daily practices build the neural pathway that makes the pause available when the amygdala fires and the carrot cake is right there.

E — Execute

The fourth step is where C.O.P.E. becomes real.

Everything before this step is insight. Clarifying what is happening. Observing where it lives in the body. Pausing to create the space. All of it is preparation. Valuable, essential preparation. But it does not take life until you do something.

Before I talk about what Execute looks like in practice, I want to give you a different way to think about the moments when you do not execute perfectly. Because this reframe may be the most important thing in this entire chapter.

My father loved old movies. Westerns especially. One of his favorites was the ones where a group of families loaded everything they owned into a line of covered wagons and set out across the frontier to stake a claim on something new. You have heard the phrase "falling off the wagon."

I want you to hear what that phrase does to the person who says it. Picture it literally. There is a family on a wagon moving out west. A young boy is sitting on the back, whittling on a piece of wood, minding his own business. The wagon hits a bump. He falls off. And no one on the wagon notices he is gone.

For the rest of the movie, you watch this boy running behind the wagon, trying to catch up. Sometimes he gets close. His hand almost reaches the back of the wagon. And then it moves a little faster, or the road turns, and he is chasing it again.

That is the story most people are living with their health. Feeling like they are always behind. Always chasing. Always just out of reach of the thing they need. It is a defeating story. It puts all the power outside of you.

I want to give you a different story. Same era. Same boy. But this time he is on a stage coach.

The stage coach is moving and it comes to a town. The boy looks around. He sees something interesting. He looks out and says: I'm going to get off here. And he gets off. He hangs out in town as long as he wants. Because he knows that either tomorrow or next week or next month, another stage coach is coming.

And when the stage coach comes, he gets back on and keeps going.

He decided to get off. He decided when to get back on. The power stayed with him the entire time. He did not fall. He chose. And the town he visited — the detour, the interruption, the imperfect week — was part of the journey, not evidence that the journey had failed.

When you eat the carrot cake, you did not fall off anything. You got off the stage coach for a moment. You looked around the town. And when you are ready, you get back on. The stage coach is still running. It will come back for you. What matters is that you get back on — and that you carry the power to make that decision rather than waiting to be rescued.

Now — back to Execute.

Execute means taking intentional action. Not just forming an intention. Acting. Because the action is what makes this real. The action is what rewires the brain. Every time you execute — even imperfectly, even incompletely, even while still feeling the pull of the original trigger — you are putting another notch in breaking the cycle. You are building a different pathway.

Here are the tools that make Execute possible:

Start small. This is not a small idea. The brain takes the path of least resistance. If the healthy choice requires significant effort and the buffering choice is right there, the buffering choice wins most of the time. Starting small means reducing the friction on the healthy side. Do not tell yourself you have to go for a thirty-minute walk. Tell yourself to put on your shoes. Just the shoes. That is the action. Because once the shoes are on and you are standing at the door, the walk becomes possible in a way it was not when you were still on the couch.

Prepare the environment before the moment arrives. This is the highest- leverage Execute tool available to you. When you are feeling calm, when the amygdala is quiet, when you have the capacity to make clear decisions — that is when you design your environment for the moment when you will not have that capacity. Fill the space with what you want to reach for. Remove what you know you will reach for when the trigger fires. You cannot design the environment in the middle of the crisis. You design it beforehand so that when the crisis comes, the environment does the work for you.

Accountability. The most reliable thing that stops me from a buffering behavior is knowing someone is watching. I had a container of what I call hump cookies in my office — they are exceptional and you probably know what I am talking about if you live in this area. I wanted to throw them away because I was doing a show that night about cleaning up your environment. I knew that if I kept them, I was going to eat them. And I knew that the community was going to hear about it. That awareness — not willpower, awareness — was what moved the cookies.

Reflect on your why. There is a young man at my house who is growing. I want to be present for him. I want to be there. The way I was going before — 285 pounds, A1C above 14, hiding the disease that was shortening my life — the time I would have had with him was getting shorter. Whenever I think about that, there is a part of me that feels something real. Not guilt. Clarity. My why is not a motivational poster. It is a specific face, a specific future I am building toward, a specific reason that reaches past the carrot cake.

Habit stacking. Link the new behavior to something you already do. After dinner, I walk. Not because I decided each evening to walk. Because I made the connection once and now one follows the other automatically. The existing habit carries the new one.

If-then planning. Before the moment arrives, decide what you will do when specific triggers fire. If I feel angry, I will take two deep breaths. If I feel frustrated, I will walk for two minutes. If I feel bored at night, I will drink a glass of water and wait five minutes. You are not making these decisions in the moment. You are making them in advance, when the prefrontal cortex is available to participate. Then when the trigger fires, the brain does not have to deliberate. It already knows.

After you execute — after the moment has passed and you have done something, anything, in the direction of the aligned choice — you evaluate.

Not judge. Evaluate.

Did the action help manage the emotion? How did you feel immediately after? What was the long-term impact of the choice? Is there anything you would do differently? What did this moment teach you about yourself?

These questions are not self-criticism. They are the learning loop that makes C.O.P.E. a system rather than a one-time intervention. Every time you run the loop and evaluate honestly, you are building the neural pathways that make the next loop faster and more reliable. The first time you do this, it will feel effortful and awkward. The tenth time, it will be faster. The fiftieth time, it will feel almost automatic.

This is neuroplasticity. Every execution — imperfect, incomplete, or clumsy — is still building something. Like my son practicing the piano, playing the whole piece even when he makes mistakes, building muscle memory that smooths the errors over time. You do not have to execute perfectly. You have to execute consistently.

Let me walk you through the full model in one real moment so you can see how it flows.

It is seven-thirty in the evening. You have had a hard day. You walk through the door depleted. A family member says something that rubs you the wrong way. The amygdala fires. You are on your way to the kitchen before the conversation has finished.

C — Clarify: What just happened? A hard day collided with a careless comment. I am not hungry. I am carrying the residue of everything that went wrong today. The comment is not the real trigger. The day is the real trigger. The comment was just the bump that knocked me off the back of the wagon.

O — Observe: One breath. Scan the body. Shoulders tight. Chest a little heavy. Breathing shallow. This is stress and exhaustion. Name it: I am tired and frustrated and a little lonely in a way I do not have words for yet. Acknowledge it: this is present, it is valid, and I do not have to fix it with food right now.

P — Pause: Four seconds in. Hold two. Four seconds out. Step away from the kitchen. Find five things in the room. Hear the sounds of the house. Thirty seconds. That is all.

E — Execute: The shoes are already by the door from this morning. Put them on. Step outside for three minutes. Or call someone from the community. Or sit with the journal for five minutes and write the actual words for what this day was. Or — if this is genuinely the right choice for this specific evening — eat something from the list, eat it slowly, eat it with awareness rather than avoidance. Because C.O.P.E. is not about never eating in the evenings. It is about choosing rather than drifting.

One final thing before we move on.

C.O.P.E. was built in the context of emotional eating and metabolic health. But the four steps work in any domain where the automatic brain overrides the intentional one. The conversation that escalates because no one paused. The financial decision made from fear. The relationship response that came from history rather than presence. The parenting moment that happened on autopilot.

Clarify what is actually happening. Observe where it lives in the body. Pause long enough for the intentional self to rejoin the conversation. Execute the designed response rather than the default one.

Two Kinds of Hunger. Two Different Responses.

C.O.P.E. was built to interrupt the automatic reach — the drift toward food that is driven by habit, emotion, access, and taste. For most people in most moments, it works exactly as described. But if you have type 2 diabetes, you are carrying a second kind of hunger that is different in origin and different in what it needs from you.

The first hunger is conditioned — the signal that fires at a familiar time, in a familiar place, in response to a familiar feeling. It is a learned pattern. It is also the hunger that C.O.P.E. was designed for. Water, wait, clarify, observe, pause, execute. Most conditioned hunger softens within ten to fifteen minutes.

The second hunger is polyphagia — the clinical symptom described in Chapter Five. It is generated not by habit but by the broken biology of the disease itself: cells that cannot absorb glucose firing a starvation signal, hormones that will not turn off, a hypothalamus that can no longer integrate the signals telling it you have eaten enough. This hunger does not soften in ten minutes. It does not respond to waiting. And here is the part that matters most for what you do next: it is simultaneously dismantling the very part of your brain you would normally use to resist it.

You cannot think your way through a signal that is degrading your ability to think. Which means the response to polyphagia cannot be a cognitive one. It has to be physical and it has to be decided before the moment arrives.

Here is how you know which signal you are dealing with. When hunger fires — whether during a fasting window or between meals — do this: drink a full glass of water and wait ten minutes. If the hunger softens, it is conditioned hunger. Run C.O.P.E. If it does not soften — or if it worsens, especially after a meal you have just finished — that is likely polyphagia. That is the disease. And the answer is not to feed it.

This is where the if-then planning tool from earlier in this chapter becomes essential — and where it must be used differently. When your prefrontal cortex is fully available, when you are calm and clear and nowhere near the moment of the signal, you make the decision in advance: if polyphagia fires, I will walk. Not "I will think about my options." Not "I will try to ride it out." A single physical action, already chosen. Shoes on. Door open. Move.

A single bout of movement restores postprandial fullness in patients with type 2 diabetes independently of every other mechanism. It addresses the disease signal at the layer where the signal is generated. And because you have pre-decided it — at a moment when your brain was fully capable of deciding — you do not have to make that choice again when your brain is not.

But here is what you must understand about the pre-decision: it only works if the walk is already familiar. A response you have never practiced is not available to you when your prefrontal cortex is compromised. The after-meal walk you are building as a daily habit — the one described in Pillar One and reinforced throughout Chapter Seven — is not only a metabolic tool. Every time you take that walk when you are not in crisis, you are loading the response that will be available to you when you are. You are practicing now so that the body knows what to do later, when the mind may not be able to lead.

C.O.P.E. for the conditioned signal. Walk — pre-decided, already practiced — for the disease signal. Two different answers for two different problems. You now have both.

This is not a diabetes tool. It is a human tool. It works wherever the gap between trigger and action exists and matters.

C.O.P.E. works best inside an environment that supports it.

Because the framework operates in the gap between trigger and action — and the size of that gap is determined in large part by what surrounds you. If the trigger is everywhere and the healthy alternative is nowhere, you are asking C.O.P.E. to do all the work. It can do some of that work. But it was not designed to work alone.

The environment is the next layer. And it is the subject of the next chapter.

CHAPTER TEN

Designing Your Environment

"You cannot out-discipline a bad environment. But you can design a good one."

I kept a bar of Cadbury chocolate in my freezer.

If you know, you know. There is something about that specific chocolate — the way it breaks, the way it melts slowly when it is frozen — that my nervous system has catalogued as a reward. And I know — with the kind of certainty that comes from years of honest self-observation — that if it is within reach when I am tired or stressed or ending a long clinic day, I am going to eat it. Not because I lack willpower. Because it is there and I am human and the amygdala does not negotiate.

One evening I was preparing an episode about environment design. I looked at that chocolate in the freezer and I made a decision. I moved it somewhere harder to reach — not because I was in danger of eating it in that moment. I did it because I understood something that has taken me years to fully internalize:

The decision about whether to eat the chocolate is not made when the chocolate is in front of me. It is made when I decide what to keep in my space and where to keep it.

This chapter is about that earlier decision.

We have spent the previous chapters building a framework for what to do when the trigger fires — how to clarify, observe, pause, and execute in the moment. That framework is essential. But it is asking you to make a high- quality decision under the worst possible conditions: tired, stressed, cortisol elevated, amygdala active, and the food right there.

Environment design is what happens before the trigger fires. It is the work you do when you are calm, clear, and capable of good decisions — work that shapes what options are available to you when you are none of those things.

You cannot out-discipline a bad environment. The research on this is consistent and clear. Willpower is a limited resource that depletes over the course of a day. Decision fatigue is real. The person who has to make fifteen food decisions by the time they walk through the door at seven o'clock in the evening has significantly less cognitive and emotional capacity for those decisions than they had at seven in the morning. And the environment — what is in the kitchen, what is on the counter, what is visible when they open the pantry — will make most of those decisions for them whether they intended it to or not.

Here is what we know about how environment shapes behavior.

The brain is a prediction machine. Its job is to anticipate what will happen next based on pattern recognition, and then to push you toward the behavior that has worked before. When the brain is in a familiar environment, it activates the behavioral patterns associated with that environment — automatically, before the conscious mind has had a chance to deliberate.

This is why you reach for something in the kitchen without deciding to. The kitchen is the cue. The reaching is the pattern. The food is the reward the pattern has been reinforced by hundreds of previous times. The behavior is not a decision. It is a prediction playing out.

Food engineers have spent decades studying this. The placement of products in grocery stores is not accidental. Eye-level shelves hold the items with the highest impulse-purchase rates. Checkout lanes are lined with small, affordable, high-sugar items specifically because people waiting in line are in a mildly depleted state and less able to override the automatic reach. The distance between desire and action has been engineered to be as small as possible.

Your home, your workplace, your car, your daily routes — these are also environments that have been shaped, mostly unconsciously, over years. The bowl of candy on the kitchen counter. The chips in the pantry at eye level. The vending machine between your desk and the bathroom. The drive- through on the route you take home every day. Each of these is a cue embedded in your environment that activates a behavioral pattern before you have made any conscious choice.

Environment design means making those choices deliberately and in advance — shaping the cues so that the automatic behavior that follows is the one you actually want.

Designing Your Home Environment

The kitchen is the most important room in your metabolic life. Not because of what you cook there, but because of what you store there and where you store it.

The research on this is striking in its specificity. Research published in a peer-reviewed journal found that women who kept fruit on the kitchen counter weighed an average of thirteen pounds less than those who did not. Those who kept cereal on the counter weighed an average of twenty pounds more. The food that is visible and accessible is the food that gets eaten — not because people are weak but because visibility is a cue and cues activate behavior.

Here is the principle: make the healthy choice the visible choice and the easy choice. Make the less healthy choice invisible and inconvenient.

This does not mean you can never have anything in your house that is not what you would typically choose. It means that the foods you want to reach for when the amygdala is running the show are the foods that are on the counter, at eye level, already washed and cut and ready. The foods you want to eat less frequently are in the back of the pantry, behind something else, requiring a deliberate decision to access.

The counter is prime real estate. What lives there should be what you want to eat. A bowl of fruit. A container of nuts. Water. If the counter holds chips and cookies and the candy someone brought over two weeks ago that you have been eating one piece at a time since then, the counter is working against you every single day.

The refrigerator follows the same logic. What is at eye level when you open it? What requires you to move things to find it? Protein and vegetables should be prepared, stored, and visible. The default meal — the thing you eat when you have no bandwidth for decisions — should be the easiest thing to find.

The pantry is where the longest-lasting decisions get made. If it does not come into the house, it cannot be eaten in a moment of weakness. This is not restriction. It is architecture. You are not depriving yourself of chips in a moment of craving. You are making the decision about chips in a moment of clarity, at the grocery store, before the craving exists.

The Grocery Store as an Environmental Decision

Every trip to the grocery store is an environment design session. What you bring home shapes what is available to you for the next week. And you make the grocery store trip when you are in a relatively regulated state — which means you have access to your prefrontal cortex in a way you will not have at ten o'clock on a Wednesday night after a difficult day.

Never shop hungry. This is not a cliché. It is neuroscience. Hunger activates the amygdala, which activates the automatic behavioral patterns associated with food seeking, which dramatically increases the likelihood of impulse purchases. The person who shops hungry brings home a different pantry than the person who shops fed.

Shop with a list built from your default meals. Not aspirational meals — the things you would cook if you had two hours and full energy. Default meals — the things you actually make on a Tuesday evening when everyone is tired. Build the list around those. Buy the ingredients. Do not buy what is not on the list unless you can immediately articulate which meal it belongs to.

The perimeter of most grocery stores contains the whole foods: produce, protein, dairy, eggs. The interior aisles contain the processed and packaged foods. This is not an accident. Shop the perimeter first and spend the majority of your time there. Enter the interior aisles with specific purpose and a specific list.

Designing Your Workplace Environment

You spend more of your waking hours at work than almost anywhere else. And the workplace environment is often one of the least intentionally designed spaces in a person's metabolic life.

The desk candy bowl is the single most underestimated environmental threat in most workplaces. It is there because someone is generous and wants the office to feel welcoming. It is accessed dozens of times a day by people who did not decide to eat — they simply walked past and their hand moved. The solution is not to judge the person who brings the candy. The solution is to create distance between yourself and the bowl — move it off your desk, ask that it be kept in a common area, or position yourself away from it when you have a choice.

Your desk should have water. Hydration reduces false hunger signals — the brain frequently misinterprets mild dehydration as hunger, particularly in the afternoon. A water bottle on the desk is an environmental intervention. A glass of water before reaching for anything else is a simple friction- increaser that works.

Lunch is a particularly important environmental decision. Where do you eat? What are your options? Do you have something prepared, or are you dependent on whatever is available when hunger arrives? The person who leaves lunch to chance in a building full of vending machines and a drive- through visible from the parking lot is making an environmental decision — just not an intentional one.

Designing for Travel

Travel is where the best-designed home environment gets no credit, because you are no longer in it. And travel tends to arrive with the exact conditions that make environmental design most critical: disrupted sleep, time zone changes, irregular schedules, limited food options, elevated stress, and the particular vulnerability that comes from being away from routine.

The five-minute plan, which we introduced in Chapter Seven, is the foundational travel protocol. Before you leave, you identify the minimum viable version of each pillar. The five-minute movement you can do in any hotel room. The default meal that exists at virtually every airport — a protein option, a salad, something that does not require you to find a specific restaurant. The morning anchor that happens before the phone is checked and the day's agenda takes over.

The travel environment should be scouted before you arrive. What does the hotel have available for breakfast? Where are the grocery stores near the venue? What are the sit-down options that have items consistent with your approach? This research takes ten minutes and prevents the situation where you are standing in an airport at seven in the morning having not eaten, tired, slightly stressed about the upcoming presentation, and the only visible option is a croissant and a pastry case.

The snacks you travel with are an environmental decision made at home. A bag of nuts. Protein bars with minimal added sugar. The foods you actually want to eat when hunger arrives in the middle of a travel day are the foods you brought from an environment you controlled.

The Social Environment

The people around you are part of your environment. Not in a way that requires you to change your friends or police your family. In a way that requires you to understand the social dynamics of eating and build some intentional structure around them.

Food is woven into almost every social occasion in human culture. Celebrations. Gatherings. Grief. Meetings. Church. Sports events. Business lunches. Someone gets a promotion and you eat. Someone has a baby and you bring food. Someone dies and you bring food. Someone is sick and you bring food. The food is always there because food is how we express care and community. It is not going away. And trying to avoid all of it would mean avoiding most of life.

The social environment design question is not how to avoid the food. It is how to participate in social eating intentionally rather than automatically.

The strategy of eating something before you arrive at the party is not about deprivation. It is about showing up to the social occasion with your hunger managed so that the decision about what to eat is made from a place of choice rather than biological urgency. The person who arrives at the party moderately full makes different choices at the food table than the person who arrives starving.

The family dinner is one of the most important social environments to design intentionally. If the eating window you have chosen conflicts with the family dinner time, adjust the eating window. We addressed this in Chapter Seven. The framework bends to fit the life. Community is not a sacrifice to make for metabolic health. It is a component of metabolic health. The two should not be in conflict, and with thoughtful design, they do not have to be.

Community accountability is also an environmental tool. Telling someone what you are doing, joining a group that shares your goals, showing up to a community consistently — these create a social environment that supports your choices rather than undermining them. The research on this is clear: people who have social accountability for their health behaviors are significantly more likely to maintain them. Not because of shame or surveillance, but because the social environment shapes what feels normal. When the people around you are doing what you are trying to do, the behavior becomes less effortful.

Environment Design and C.O.P.E.

Let me connect environment design back to the framework we built in the last chapter, because these two tools are designed to work together.

C.O.P.E. operates in the gap between trigger and action. It gives you the tools to catch the drift, interrupt the automatic, and make an intentional choice in the moment. But the size of that gap —

how much space you have to work with between the trigger and the behavior — is determined largely by the environment.

When the trigger-food is on the counter directly in your path, the gap is essentially zero. The hand moves before the framework has had a chance to activate. When the trigger-food is not in the house, the gap is the entire trip to the store — during which C.O.P.E. has ample time to run its full sequence.

This is why I said earlier that environment design is where the earliest and most leverage-rich decisions get made. Not because C.O.P.E. does not work — it does. But it works best when the environment is not actively working against it. Stack the environment in your favor and the framework has the space it needs to operate.

This is also the reactance principle from Chapter Three working in your favor rather than against you. When the food is not in the house, you are not fighting it. You are not exercising discipline. You are simply living in a space that does not create the problem. The holly bush is still interesting. But if you cannot see it from the window, it stops being the thing you think about.

Think of it this way. C.O.P.E. is the parachute. Environment design is choosing not to jump from a plane without one. Both matter. The parachute is essential. But you want to make the decision about the parachute before you are in the air.

Your Environment Audit

Here is a practical starting point. Before you do anything else with the information in this chapter, conduct an honest audit of your three most important environments: your home, your workplace, and your car.

For each environment, ask three questions:

What is currently in this environment that makes the aligned choice harder? The candy bowl. The chips at eye level. The drive-through on the daily commute. The vending machine between your desk and the bathroom. These are the environmental cues that are currently working against you. Name them specifically.

What is currently missing from this environment that would make the aligned choice easier? The fruit on the counter. The prepared protein in the refrigerator. The water bottle on the desk. The planned eating options for your window already ready in the car. The default meal ingredients already bought and ready. Name these specifically too.

What is the one change I can make today — right now — that would reduce the friction between my intentions and my behavior? Not the complete overhaul. The one change. The thing that, if it existed tomorrow morning, would make tomorrow slightly more aligned than today. At the end of this book, you will find a page called Start Here. It asks this exact question in three different ways, depending on where you are. Prepare to answer it.

Start there. One change. Because the environment does not need to be perfect to be significantly better than it currently is. And a significantly better environment produces significantly better outcomes without requiring any additional willpower at all.

We have now covered the three pillars, the behavioral and emotional framework, and the environmental layer that supports them all.

You have the metabolic science. You have the tools for the moment the trigger fires. You have the design principles for shaping the environment before the trigger fires.

What remains is the larger vision. Because all of this — the fasting, the food quality, the C.O.P.E. framework, the environment design — is not the destination. It is the foundation. The question that has been waiting since the Introduction is: once your health is no longer the problem, what becomes possible?

PART FOUR

What Becomes Possible

CHAPTER ELEVEN

The People Around You

There is a question I get asked more than almost any other.

It comes from the wife of the patient. It comes from the adult daughter of the mother. It comes from the husband, the brother, the son, the friend, the pastor, the woman in the third pew who has been watching her best friend's blood sugar climb for three years and does not know what to do anymore.

The question is some version of this:

How do I get through to them?

The husband whose wife will not stop the bread. The daughter whose mother turns off the continuous glucose monitor when it alarms at the dinner table. The son whose father has been told for fifteen years to walk and has not walked. The friend whose friend has stopped coming to lunch because the lunch is the conversation.

How do I get through to them?

I want to tell you something I have learned over twenty-something years of being asked that question.

It is the wrong question.

Not because the people asking it are wrong to be asking. They are asking out of love. They are asking out of fear. They are asking because they have watched someone they care about fight a disease for years and lose ground, and they cannot stand it anymore, and they do not know what else to do. The asking is good. The asking is the evidence of a love that is still trying.

The question itself is wrong because of what is hidden inside it.

Hidden inside *how do I get through to them* is an assumption: that what is needed is the right delivery of something they already know. The right tone. The right moment. The right sentence. As if the patient with diabetes simply has not yet heard the message, and once it lands cleanly, they will respond.

But that is not the situation.

The patient has heard the message. Hundreds of times. From doctors. From spouses. From children. From their own internal voice every time they look at a number they do not want to see. The message is not what is missing.

What is missing is a language they can hear it in.

—

I want to show you what I mean.

Imagine a mother and her adult daughter. The mother has type 2 diabetes. She has been managing it, in the loose sense of that word, for years. She wears a continuous glucose monitor. Sometimes it alarms. Sometimes the number goes high after dinner and the device buzzes from her arm and the family hears it across the room.

The daughter looks over.

The mother reaches down and turns it off.

The daughter, who loves her mother, who has watched her mother's blood sugar climb for years, who has read articles and watched videos and tried to be informed, says something she has said a hundred times before.

Mom, you have to eat differently.

The mother does not look up.

The daughter says it again, a little sharper.

Mom, the device went off because your sugar is too high. You have to take this seriously.

The mother sets her fork down. The energy in the room changes. The husband at the end of the table puts his head down. The grandchildren get quiet. And the mother says something that will end the conversation but not solve anything:

I know what I am doing.

She does not know what she is doing. She knows that. The daughter knows that. But the words came out anyway, because what the mother is actually saying underneath those words is something else entirely. What she is actually saying is: please stop. I cannot bear another one of these conversations. I have been trying. I have been failing. And every time you say it I feel like a child who is being scolded for something that is breaking my heart.

The daughter does not hear that. The daughter hears refusal.

So the daughter goes home and calls her sister and says I do not know how to get through to mom. And the next week we sit across the table and it happens again. And again. And the mother gets a little quieter. And the daughter gets a little louder. And the disease, meanwhile, continues to do what the disease does.

That is the wrong question producing its predictable result.

The right question is not how do I get through to them.

The right question is: what is the language this person can actually hear me in?

—

I want to tell you what is happening inside the person who is being spoken to in the wrong language.

The patient hears the daughter's words — *eat differently, take this seriously* — and a chemistry kicks off underneath the surface that is not the chemistry of receiving information. It is the chemistry of being judged. It is the chemistry of being a child again. It is the chemistry of the whole accumulated weight of every doctor's appointment, every disappointing number, every time they tried and failed, every time they were told they were not doing enough. And that chemistry has only one direction it knows how to go.

It goes inward.

The patient pulls back. The patient gets quiet. The patient turns the monitor off. The patient stops mentioning the appointment. The patient becomes harder to reach, not easier — not because they do not love the person speaking to them, but because the speaking itself has begun to hurt.

A patient told me a story once that I have not forgotten.

She was seventy-six years old. Her husband had come home from the grocery store, and he could not find her. The house was quiet. Her car was in the driveway. He called her name. She did not answer. He went room to room. Eventually he came to the bathroom and the door was closed. He opened the door. The bathroom was empty. But the shower curtain was drawn.

He pulled it back.

His seventy-six-year-old wife, fully clothed, was standing in the shower eating a Snickers bar.

She had heard him come home. She had not wanted him to fuss at her. So she had taken the candy bar into the bathroom and stepped into the shower and pulled the curtain closed, hoping he would not look there.

I want you to understand what happened in that house. That is not a story about a woman who did not love her husband. That is not a story about a woman who did not care about her health. That is a story about a person whose disease had gone into hiding because the people around her had made the disease impossible to talk about.

She loved him. He loved her. They had been married for decades. And there she was, fully clothed in the shower, eating a Snickers bar in secret, because the alternative — being caught eating it in the kitchen — was worse than hiding from the man who had been asking her for years to do better.

That is what the wrong language does, given enough time. It does not just fail to reach the patient. It pushes the disease into the dark. And what lives in the dark grows.

—

So what is the right language?

I want to describe a moment that happens regularly in my exam room. When a couple comes in together and I can feel the friction between them — when one of them is frustrated and the other is defensive, when the spouse is exasperated and the patient has gone quiet — I do something before we talk about blood sugar.

I have them switch positions in the room. I ask the spouse to come around to the patient's side. I ask them to put their hands on the patient's shoulders, or to take the patient's hand. And I ask them to say, by name, one sentence.

I know that managing diabetes is difficult.

That is the whole sentence. No qualifier. No *but*. No pivot to what the patient should be doing instead. No preamble about all the things they have been worried about. Just that. *I know that managing diabetes is difficult.*

I ask them to say it slowly. I ask them to mean it.

And I tell them: after you say that sentence — after you say it and let it be heard — you are then free to say anything else you want. Anything. You can express your worry. You can ask for changes. You can have whatever conversation you have been waiting to have. But you have to start there.

I have watched the moment land more times than I can count.

The spouse says it. The patient hears it. Something shifts in the room that is almost physical. Because what has almost always been missing from those conversations is exactly that — the acknowledgment that the patient has been trying, that the disease is hard, that the fact of not having succeeded does not mean the patient has not been working. The fussing the spouse has been doing for years has not been carrying that acknowledgment. The fussing has been carrying fear. But because nobody has named the fear as fear, the patient has only been able to receive it as judgment.

The fussing is fear wearing anger's clothes.

When the acknowledgment lands first — when the patient hears *I know that this is difficult* before they hear anything else — the rest of what the spouse has to say can land on a different surface. It is not landing on a person who feels judged. It is landing on a person who feels seen. A person who feels seen can hear things that a person who feels judged cannot.

Then I ask the patient to do something in return.

I ask the patient to take the spouse's hand and say, also by name:

Thank you for caring about me. I give you permission to speak into my life about my health.

That second sentence is the one that changes everything.

Because what it does is it transforms the relationship. It moves the spouse from being perceived as a warden into being explicitly invited as a partner. The patient has, in their own words, granted access. The conversation that follows is no longer surveillance. It is participation. It is two people who want the same thing, who have just said so to each other in a language the other can finally hear.

—

I want to be clear about what is happening at a deeper level when this exercise works.

It is not that the words are magic. It is not that *I know that managing diabetes is difficult* is a special incantation. The words are doing something specific: they are translating fear back into the language it actually is.

The spouse has been carrying fear for a long time. Fear of losing the person they love. Fear of watching the disease take pieces of them. Fear of waking up one day and finding out the warning signs have become the diagnosis they could not undo. That fear has been coming out as policing. As fussing. As nagging. As the running commentary at the dinner table. The fear has been there the whole time. It has just been wearing clothes that the patient could not recognize.

When the spouse says *I know that managing diabetes is difficult,* what they are doing is taking off the anger costume the fear has been wearing. They are letting the fear show up as itself. And fear, shown as fear, is one of the most powerful things one human being can offer another. It says: I am scared because I love you. It says: I cannot stand to lose you. It says: I have been ugly about this because I have been desperate, not because I think you are weak.

The patient can receive that. The patient has been waiting, often for years, to receive exactly that.

The same dynamic operates in every relationship in which someone with diabetes has been receiving the wrong language. The mother and the adult daughter. The father and the son. The pastor and the parishioner. The friend and the friend.

The instruction is the same. Find the fear under the speech. Name it. And before you say anything else — acknowledge.

—

I want to say one more thing about who else is in the room.

This chapter has been talking about close relationships — the ones where the disease is being talked about every day. But there is a wider circle around every patient with diabetes that has its own version of the wrong language, and I do not want to leave that out.

There is the church community where the disease is treated as a moral failing.

There is the workplace where the patient feels they have to hide the appointments.

There is the friend group that organizes itself around food the patient cannot eat in the proportions everybody else is eating it.

There is the doctor's office — and I include myself in this — where for decades the language has been *compliance* and *non-compliance,* a vocabulary that turns the patient into a moral subject rather than a person with a body responding to conditions.

Every one of those settings has its own wrong language, and every one of them is fixable in essentially the same way. Find the fear, the anxiety, or the unstated expectation underneath the words. Acknowledge first. Speak from where you actually are, not from the script the situation has handed you.

The diabetic in your life does not need more information.

They need to feel safe enough to say what they have not been able to say.

And the people around the person with diabetes do not need a sharper way to deliver the message.

They need a softer doorway to walk through.

—

If you are the person with diabetes and you have been on the receiving end of the wrong language for a long time, I want you to hear this.

You can teach them.

You can hand them this chapter and say *this is the language I have been waiting for you to use with me.* You can tell them, in your own words, what it has felt like to be on the receiving end of fear dressed up as anger. You can say what you wish they had said. You can ask them, plainly, to start with the acknowledgment. People who love you will, in my experience, almost always rise to that ask once it is named clearly.

And if you are the person who has been speaking the wrong language — if you have been the daughter at the dinner table, the husband in the kitchen, the friend in the third pew — I want you to hear this.

You were not failing.

You were loving someone with a disease nobody had taught you the language for. The fussing came from love. The fear came from love. The lectures came from love. None of that was wrong. What was wrong was the language they were arriving in.

You can change the language. You do not have to change the love.

—

Diabetes is not a disease that lives in one body.

It lives between people. It lives in the silence between the mother and the daughter at the dinner table. It lives in the bathroom shower where the candy bar gets eaten in secret. It lives in the marriage where one person has stopped saying anything about it because the saying has stopped helping.

The exit is not just metabolic. The exit is also relational.

When the people around you can finally meet you with the language you can actually hear, the disease loses one of its most powerful allies — the isolation it has been feeding on. And when you can finally hear them as the frightened, loving people they have been all along, you lose one of your most powerful obstacles — the wall between you and the support that has been there the entire time, just speaking in a language you could not receive.

Build the new language.

It is one of the most consequential things you will do in this work. And the principle is the same one that has been running through this entire book. You do not fix what is broken between you and the people who love you with willpower. You fix it the way you fix anything that matters — with a design. A small one, in this case. Two sentences. Said in the right order, by both people, before any other conversation happens.

That is the entire intervention. It is structural, like everything else in this framework. It works not because anyone is trying harder. It works because the structure makes the better conversation easier than the worse one.

I know that this is difficult.

Start there.

The rest follows.

That is the subject of the next chapter.

CHAPTER TWELVE

What Becomes Possible — And How to Hold It

I want to return to a patient you met briefly in Chapter One.

Her name is Sandra. She is sixty-three years old. She is a hospital administrator — one of the most organized, disciplined, capable people I have ever met. She has carried type 2 diabetes for eleven years. She has been on three medications. Her A1C, on her best months, hovers in the high 7s. On her worst, it climbs above 9.

She came to me already exhausted. She had been doing what was asked of her for over a decade — the appointments, the prescriptions, the conversations about her numbers, the slow accumulation of tools that managed the disease without ever making it smaller.

I want to tell you what changed for Sandra once the gap finally started to close — once we had the right tools in place and the framework she was living inside of stopped working against her. I want to tell you about the first time her A1C fell below 7 in eleven years. About the medications we have started removing. About the granddaughter she can now keep up with on a walk to the park. About the weight that came off and stayed off because the conditions had finally changed underneath it.

But before I tell you any of that, I want to tell you something else.

Sandra is not a patient.

Sandra is a pattern.

She is your mom. She is your dad. She is your cousin who keeps showing up to the family Thanksgiving with a new prescription and the same tired explanation about how the doctor is adjusting things again. She is the woman in your church who has been quietly managing her blood sugar for fifteen years and has not once been told that anything else was possible.

She is you. If you are reading this book, she is you.

And she is me.

I want you to hold that for a moment. Because the temptation when you read a story about a patient who got better is to put her on the other side of a wall — the patient over there, you over here, her victory the kind of thing that happens to other people in other circumstances with other resources and other capabilities. That wall is part of what has been keeping you sick.

The wall is not real.

There is no separate population of people for whom the exit was always going to be possible. There is no special category of patient who gets to leave. There is the framework, and there is everyone who picks it up.

Sandra picked it up. And once she did, the same biology that had been working against her for eleven years began working with her. Not because she became someone different. Because the conditions she lived inside of finally matched what her body had been asking for the whole time.

What follows in this chapter is the territory she walked into, and what almost every patient I have walked through this work has eventually found waiting for them on the other side. I want you to read it not as someone else's reward. I want you to read it as a description of what the exit actually looks like once you reach it.

Because Sandra is the pattern.

And the pattern is yours.

I ask every patient the same question when they come back after their first real progress.

Not what their A1C is. Not how much weight they have lost. Not which medication we are reducing or eliminating. Those numbers matter and we review them. But first I ask:

What has surprised you most?

And almost universally, the answer is not about the numbers.

I think of a patient who had been living with diabetes for nine years when he came to me. Nine years of medications, of quarterly appointments, of a blood sugar that hovered just out of control no matter what he adjusted. When he came back after his first four months in the framework, his A1C had dropped from 9.2 to 6.8. He had lost twenty-seven pounds. We were reducing his second medication. By every clinical measure, the appointment was a success.

I asked him what had surprised him most.

He sat quietly for a moment and then said: I forgot what it felt like to feel good. I had been feeling bad for so long that I thought that was just what I felt like. I thought that was me.

He was not talking about his blood sugar. He was talking about who he had been living as for nine years — a person whose body was a problem to be managed, whose daily experience was shaped by fatigue and fog and the low-level depletion of a metabolism running chronically off-course. He had normalized an existence that was significantly diminished from what he was capable of. And he had normalized it so completely that he had forgotten there was anything else.

That is what I hear most often when I ask the surprise question. Not surprise at the numbers. Surprise at the return of something the patient had stopped expecting to find.

They tell me they got back a feeling of control.

That for years — sometimes decades — they had felt like passengers in their own health, watching the disease do what it was going to do, managing consequences rather than shaping outcomes. And now, for the first time, they feel like they are the ones making decisions. The framework gave them something that no prescription ever had: agency. The sense that what they do matters. That the disease is responsive to their choices. That they are not trapped inside a condition that will simply progress regardless of how they live.

They tell me their self-esteem has returned. That they had quietly, over time, come to see themselves as people who could not do what needed to be done. People who knew what to eat and did not eat it. People who understood what the disease required and could not deliver it. That identity — the failing patient — had settled into their sense of self in a way that reached far beyond their bloodwork. And now that identity is loosening. They are not a person who failed at diabetes management. They are a person who never had the right design.

They tell me the energy came back. The physical energy, often dramatically. The mental energy. The emotional energy. The energy that had been consumed for years by fighting their own biology, managing their own shame, and carrying the low-level exhaustion of a body running on chronic hyperinsulinemia and chronic cortisol. When the metabolism stabilizes, when the blood sugar stops spiking and crashing through the day, when the insulin finally has the recovery time it needs — the person who comes out the other side has reserves they had forgotten they possessed.

These are not clinical outcomes.

They are identity outcomes. And they are, in my experience, the most important thing that happens when someone reverses their diabetes.

The A1C is the evidence. The identity shift is the thing itself.

Relationships

Chronic illness affects relationships in ways that rarely get discussed in a clinical setting. The person whose blood sugar is unstable is also a person whose mood is unstable — because blood sugar and mood are not separate systems. The glucose crash at three in the afternoon is also an irritability event. The chronic fatigue of hyperinsulinemia is also a withdrawal from presence. The shame of the disease — the hiding, the silence, the not wanting to explain why you are eating differently or checking your glucose at the restaurant table — creates a kind of emotional distance that compounds over time.

I think of a man who came to me whose wife had finally said something to him that he could not dismiss. She told him she felt like she was living with a stranger. Not because he was unkind. Because he was not there. He was physically present at dinner, at family events, on weekends. But the version of him that arrived was always running at partial capacity — distracted, short-tempered in the afternoon, exhausted by eight o'clock, disappearing into himself in the hours when their family was actually together.

He had attributed it to stress. To work. To the ordinary pressures of middle age. He had not connected it to the blood sugar that was swinging through the day, to the cortisol load of a metabolism running chronically off-course, to the particular emotional dulling that comes with years of hyperinsulinemia.

Six months after beginning the framework, his wife told me — at a follow-up appointment he had asked her to attend — that her husband had come back. Not without difficulty. But substantially. The afternoons were different. He was present at dinner in a way he had not been in years. The stranger had not fully disappeared, but the man she had married was recognizable again.

When the metabolic system stabilizes, the emotional system often follows. One of the primary physiological drivers of mood dysregulation has been removed. The person who is no longer riding a blood sugar roller coaster through the day is, in a measurable and real sense, a more available person. More present. More regulated. More able to show up for the people who matter to them.

Physical Capacity

The body that is metabolically healthy is a body that can do more. This sounds obvious but the implications run deeper than most people realize until they experience the change.

Chronic inflammation — which hyperinsulinemia drives — affects joint health, recovery time, sleep quality, and the basic physical experience of inhabiting a body. People who have been living with chronic metabolic disease often do not know how much physical discomfort they have normalized until it is gone. The joint pain they attributed to aging. The sleep that never felt fully restorative. The physical heaviness that had become so familiar it felt like personality.

One of my patients told me at a six-month follow-up that he had started playing basketball again. He had played seriously in his twenties, had given it up in his thirties as his weight climbed and his joints stopped cooperating, and had quietly accepted that part of his life as finished. He was in his mid- fifties when he came to me. Four months into the framework, he had lost thirty-one pounds and his knee pain — which he had been managing with anti-inflammatories for years — had largely resolved.

He walked into my exam room that day and said: I played basketball on Saturday. I had not played in fifteen years.

He was not describing a fitness achievement. He was describing the return of something he had grieved without quite naming it as a loss. Physical capacity is not just about exercise metrics. It is about the texture of your life — what you can participate in, what you can offer to the people you love, what remains available to you as you move through your days. The grandparent who can get on the floor and play. The parent who can throw a ball in the yard. The person who can climb the stairs, carry their groceries, travel without their health being the primary logistical challenge of the trip. These are not trivial things. They are the substance of a life fully inhabited.

Unlimited potential does not mean the absence of limits. It means the removal of the ones that were never supposed to be there.

These are the returns on the exit. Not just the number. The return of the person — the capacity the disease had been consuming, now available for everything else. And it raises the question this chapter was always building toward: what does it take to hold what you have found?

Because the exit is not a single event. The life you have reclaimed has to be designed to sustain it.

There is a pattern I have watched play out hundreds of times in my practice.

A patient comes in for a follow-up. Their numbers are dramatically better. A1C down. Weight down. Medications reduced or eliminated. They are energized, focused, proud of what they have accomplished. We talk about what they did. They describe the changes they made with the kind of clarity and conviction that only comes from having lived through something real.

Then I ask the question that matters most at this stage:

What are you going to do when life gets hard again?

Not if. When.

Because the diagnosis did not arrive during the easiest season of their life. The metabolic disease developed over years inside a life that was already full of demands, relationships, obligations, seasons of grief and seasons of celebration, the ordinary relentlessness of being a person in the world. The framework helped them find their way through. But the life did not pause while they did the work. And it will not pause now that the work is showing results.

The question is not how to maintain perfect adherence. The question is how to build a life that holds your health even when everything around it is in motion. Not a rigid structure that shatters when circumstances change. A living architecture that flexes with the life and returns to alignment when it drifts.

Let me tell you why most people fail to maintain what they have gained.

It is not because they stop caring. It is not because the knowledge disappears. It is not because the disease reasserts itself with some new force they cannot resist.

It is because they were running on motivation.

Motivation is a powerful starting fuel. It responds to novelty, to visible progress, to the excitement of early results. The first significant lab improvement. The first week of consistent fasting. The first time someone asks if you have lost weight and you say yes and mean it. Motivation is real and valuable and completely unreliable as a long-term energy source.

Motivation fades. Not because you are weak. Because that is what motivation does. The novelty wears off. The progress slows as the early gains stabilize. Life reasserts its demands and the mental bandwidth that was available for the new behaviors gets redistributed to everything else. And the person who built their health on motivation finds themselves back at the beginning, wondering what happened to the person who was doing so well.

The person who built their health on structure finds themselves still moving forward.

Structure is the difference between a decision you make every day and a decision you made once.

When you decide every morning whether to walk, you are asking your prefrontal cortex to expend decision-making energy before the day has even begun. Some mornings it says yes. Some mornings — when you are tired, when the schedule is already full, when the day is making demands before it has properly started — it says not today. Over time, the not-today mornings accumulate and the habit erodes.

When walking is a non-negotiable — when it is not a decision but a given, as fixed and unconsidered as brushing your teeth — the prefrontal cortex does not get consulted. It simply happens. The decision was made once, weeks or months ago, and it has been executed daily since. The behavior is anchored to structure rather than to motivation, and structure does not have bad days.

This is what I mean when I say that people do not fail because they lack desire or vision or even knowledge. They fail because they lack structure. Because the healthy behavior was something they were trying to do rather than something they had decided they were.

Monitoring

Sustainable metabolic health requires ongoing measurement. Not obsessive measurement. Regular, honest, informed measurement that tells you what is actually happening in your body rather than what you hope or fear is happening.

The continuous glucose monitor is one of the most powerful real-time feedback tools available for metabolic health. It shows you what your food choices actually do to your blood sugar — not what the glycemic index says they should do, what they actually do in your body, on this day, under these conditions. It shows you what stress does to your glucose. What sleep deprivation does. What a walk does. What the carrot cake does. The data is not a verdict. It is information. And information, honestly used, makes every subsequent decision smarter.

The A1C is the long-game measurement. It tells you the story of the last three months — not the last three days. When the trend is moving in the right direction, it is confirmation that the structure is working. When the trend moves the wrong way, it is early warning — an invitation to examine what has shifted before the shift becomes entrenched.

I encourage everyone to approach their numbers with curiosity rather than dread. A number that has moved in the wrong direction is not a failure. It is data. It is the body reporting something about what has changed. Treat it as a diagnostic, not a verdict, and it becomes the most useful piece of information you have.

Community as a Structural Tool

I want to say something about community that goes beyond the standard advice about finding a support group.

Community is not a motivational tool. It is a structural one.

When you are part of a community that shares your goals and your values, the healthy behaviors become normal. Not extraordinary. Not requiring explanation or defense. Normal. The person who fasts among people who have never heard of fasting has to justify themselves constantly — at every meal, at every social occasion, every time someone asks why they are not eating. That constant justification is a friction cost that accumulates. The person who fasts among others who also fast has no such cost. The behavior is simply what people in this community do.

I think of a woman who came to me after years of failed attempts. She was knowledgeable, motivated, and repeatedly unsuccessful. When we looked at her pattern, what we found was that every attempt had ended at a social event — a family dinner, a work function, a celebration where she was the only one doing something different. The social friction of being the exception had worn her down every time.

She joined the online community that had grown around the work I do. Within two months, something had shifted. She told me at her next appointment: these people fast like I fast. They talk about blood sugar the way I think about blood sugar. When I'm having a hard day, I can tell people who understand what a hard day means. For the first time since starting this, I don't feel alone in it.

The change continues to hold. This is no accident. Community did not give her new information or new tools. She had the information and the tools. Community gave her a world in which her choices were normal. That changed everything.

When You Drift

You will drift. This is not a prediction of failure. It is a description of how change actually works in a real life.

There will be a season when the fasting window collapses. A week when the food choices slide back toward old patterns. A period when the cortisol load is high and the structure that held everything in place gets disrupted by a job change, a family crisis, an illness, a grief, a season of life that demands more than the structure was built for. These are not signs that the framework has failed. They are signs that you are living a full human life inside a framework that was designed to survive exactly this.

I think of a patient who had been in the framework for about seven months when his father died. He had been doing extraordinarily well — A1C below 6.5 for the first time in years, off two medications, consistent with his fasting and his movement. The grief, when it came, was not something the structure could fully absorb. He stopped fasting. He ate in ways that comforted him and ignored what they did to his glucose. He came to his next appointment apologetic, ashamed, expecting a lecture.

I told him: your father died. The framework will still be here. Let's talk about how to find your way back.

He came back. Not immediately, not perfectly, but he came back. And when he did, he brought something with him that he had not had before: the knowledge that the framework could survive a significant disruption and still be there when he was ready. That knowledge made him more secure in the framework, not less. The drift had not destroyed what he had built. It had tested it, and the foundation had held.

The stage coach is still running. It will come back for you.

What matters in the moment of drift is not the drift itself. It is the response. The person who treats a difficult week as evidence that they cannot do this — who collapses into all-or-nothing thinking, who waits for Monday, who starts over from zero with the same internal conditions that created the drift — will cycle through the same pattern indefinitely. The person who treats the drift as information — who asks what shifted, what the stress load was, what structural support was missing — gets back on the stage coach carrying something valuable. Drift is not failure. Drift is what happens when life exceeds the structure temporarily. And the response to drift is not shame. It is one structural adjustment. The anchor you have been skipping. The community check-in you stopped attending. Start there. The system will respond.

The Long View

I want to close this chapter by talking about what you are actually building.

Not a diet. Not a program. Not a challenge with a certificate at the end.

A life.

The work of this book is the work of redesigning the conditions of your daily existence so that the body you want to live in becomes the natural outcome of the life you are actually living. Not the life you are performing. Not the life you sustain through heroic effort. The life that flows from a rhythm you have chosen, an alignment you maintain honestly, and a structure you have built deliberately. That life does not require perfection. It requires direction. And direction, maintained consistently, is enough.

This is what I mean when I say health is not a destination. It is a foundation. The person who finds their exit does not arrive at a finish line where the work is over. They arrive at a starting line where the real possibilities begin. The energy that was consumed fighting the disease becomes available for living. The mental bandwidth that was devoted to managing the illness becomes available for building. The capacity that the disease had been quietly consuming — the presence, the vitality, the ability to show up fully for the people and purposes that matter — is returned.

I think about the woman who came off her last diabetes medication after thirty years and walked into my exam room and hugged me. She was sixty-three years old. She had been coming to see me for years, always with her daughter. She was not crying because her number had changed. She was crying because of what the number meant. Because after thirty years of being told the ceiling was fixed, she discovered it was not. And in that discovery was something no lab result can capture: the return of the belief that things can get better. That the body she had been fighting against was capable of becoming an ally. That the life she had been managing from inside the disease could be lived from outside it.

Thirty years. She had carried that ceiling for thirty years. And it was not the truth about what she was capable of. It was a story built from a moment in medicine when we did not yet know what we know now.

You do not have to carry your ceiling for thirty years. You have the exit now.

We do not default to our goals. We default to our design.

Design your life. Design it with rhythm and alignment and structure. Design it with the non-negotiable minimum that holds even on the worst days. Design it with the community that makes your choices normal and your hard days survivable. Design it with the monitoring that tells you the truth and the curiosity that treats the truth as information rather than verdict.

Design it, and the health will follow — consistently, in a direction that changes what is possible for you.

That is what this book has been building toward. Not a set of rules. A design. Not compliance. Identity.

The framework is complete. The exit is real. And what you build on the other side of it — that is entirely, gloriously yours.

CONCLUSION

You Have Everything You Need

"The exit exists. I found it. And I came back to show you the way out."

You know this story. I told it at the beginning of this book.

The fall in Rose Hall Town. The doctor who said there was nothing more to do. My grandmother, Rebecca, who said no. Who sat by my bedside and refused to accept that conclusion as the final word on what was possible.

I recovered. Against what the expert in the room had decided was probable.

I did not understand the full weight of what she had done until I was old enough to be told the story — that the doctor had essentially given up, and that she had not. That my recovery was not just a childhood memory. It was evidence that exits exist even when the people with credentials say they do not.

I have been looking for exits my entire life. I did not always know that was what I was doing. But when I trace the thread back through everything — the PhD that did not work, the medical school that almost did not work, the three attempts at the boards, the diagnosis that arrived in the night, the decade of hiding that followed, the raft on the river during my son's Spring Break when I finally ran out of air and let go — I can see it clearly now.

My grandmother taught me one of the most important lessons in life:

The limits you were given are not always the limits that exist.

Sometimes it is a story someone told. Sometimes it is a system that was never designed with you in mind. Sometimes it is the accumulated weight of evidence that has only ever been gathered inside the old conditions — and has never been tested against the new ones.

You have spent much of your health life inside the old conditions. This book is the beginning of the new ones.

You have the three pillars that move blood sugar. You have H.E.A.T. – the four forces that have been driving your eating beneath the level of conscious choice. You have C.O.P.E. – a framework for the moments that undo you. And you have something harder to name but more important than all of it: the understanding that your body was never broken. It was responding. Now you know what to give it instead. I want to talk not about what you have learned but about who you are becoming.

Because information alone does not change a life. You have known things for years that have not changed your life. What changes a life is when information becomes identity – when the new understanding stops being something you are trying to apply and starts being something you simply are.

That shift does not happen in a single reading. It happens in the living. In the morning you choose to walk even though it is easier not to. In the moment at the grocery store when you read the label on the seasoning blend and put it back. In the evening you sit with the difficult feeling instead of reaching for the thing that has always made it temporarily quiet. In the conversation where you tell someone what you are doing and why, and hear yourself speak it out loud as if it is simply true, because it is.

Each of those moments is not a victory over your old self. It is a decision that becomes design. The person who makes enough of those decisions – not perfectly, not without backsliding, not without the occasional Tuesday that ends with you standing in a kitchen wondering how you got there – eventually looks up and realizes the identity has shifted. Not because they tried harder. Because they kept showing up.

You are becoming someone for whom metabolic health is not a project but a foundation. Someone who fasts not as a discipline but as a rhythm. Someone who understands their own emotional triggers not as weaknesses but as information. Someone who has stopped fighting their body and started designing conditions in which it can do what it has always been capable of doing.

That person is not somewhere in your future. They are in the choices you make starting today.

Before I send you forward I want to say one more thing about the shame.

You may still be carrying some of it. That is alright. It does not have to be gone before you begin. It does not have to be resolved before the exit becomes real. Shame dissolves in motion. It does not dissolve in waiting.

The shame that kept me hiding for over two decades — that kept me from being the most useful person in the room for patients who needed exactly what I had — did not dissolve because I figured something out. It dissolved because I started telling the truth. First to one teenager and his parents. Then to my staff. Then to the community that was watching the YouTube channel I had built to talk about everything except the thing I was most qualified to talk about. Then to the tens of thousands of people who have found their way to this work because someone somewhere shared it with someone who needed it.

The truth that broke the shame was not a sophisticated truth. It was the simplest one available:

I have this disease. I was not doing a good job with it. And I was afraid of what you would think.

That is all it took. Not a perfectly managed A1C. Not a before-and-after photo. Not the credentials or the clinical expertise or the years of training. Just the honesty that I was human and struggling and afraid — the same honesty you have been carrying, in your own form, since the day the diagnosis arrived.

You do not need to be further along than you are to begin. You do not need to have it figured out. You do not need to be worthy of the exit before you walk through it.

You just need to take the next step.

So here is what I want you to do.

Pick one thing. Not the optimal thing. Not the complete overhaul. The one thing that, if you did it today, would mean that today was not a zero. The page after the conclusion will help you choose it.

Maybe it is going to bed twenty minutes earlier, because the night is where the day's stress turns into tomorrow's blood sugar. Maybe it is letting the next craving sit for ten seconds before you decide, just to prove the decision is yours. Maybe it is a ten-minute walk after dinner that begins the habit before the habit is a habit. Maybe it is reading one label. Maybe it is telling one person what you are trying to do, which is its own kind of beginning.

Do that one thing. Not because it will reverse your diabetes today. Because it will prove to you that you can move. And the person who can move can find the exit. The person who is standing still, waiting to feel ready, waiting for the perfect moment, waiting for the shame to lift before they begin — that person is still under the raft.

Let go.

Not of your food. Not of your family. Not of the life you have built. Let go of the story that the ceiling is permanent. Let go of the verdict the system handed you when it said manage it and accept the limit. Let go of the belief that you are the exception to the possibility the science has demonstrated — that you are the one person for whom the exit does not exist.

It exists. I know because I walked through it.

And on the other side is not a perfect body or a perfect life or a version of yourself who never struggles. On the other side is a foundation. Solid ground from which the rest of what you want to build becomes possible. The years with the people you love. The energy for the things that matter. The presence you have been trying to offer while the disease was quietly consuming the capacity for it.

My grandmother sat by my bedside when the doctor had already moved on. She refused the verdict. She believed in the exit before there was any evidence for it. And she passed that belief to me. I will carry it for the rest of my life.

I am passing it to you now.

The exit is real.

You were never failing.

You were never given the right design.

Now you have it.

Dwain Woode, MD

Huntsville, Alabama dwainwoode.com

START HERE

You have read the framework. The conclusion asked you to choose one thing. Here is how to decide which one.

If you were recently diagnosed or your numbers have just shifted:

Start with the fasting window. This is Pillar One — the intervention with the most direct and immediate effect on insulin. Choose a window that fits your life. Eat with your family. Close it an hour after dinner. Open it later the next morning. Hold that window for two weeks before you add anything else. The number will respond.

If you have been managing this for years and nothing is moving:

Start with one environment audit. Go to the kitchen tonight. Find the one item that you know — with complete honesty — is working against you. Move it. Not dramatically. Just further away, less visible, less automatic. That one decision, made now while you are clear, is worth more than ten decisions made in the moment when you are not. Do the audit before you go to bed.

If you are reading this for someone you love:

Start with the two sentences from Chapter Eleven. Say them. Not to fix anything. Not to start a conversation about what they should be doing differently. Just say them, and mean them. Everything else this framework asks of you as a support person follows from that.

One thing. This week. That is the whole instruction.

QUICK REFERENCE GUIDES

These tools are designed to be used in the moment — not read once and set aside. Return to them whenever you need them.

C.O.P.E. — Real-Time Behavioral Framework

Use this framework in the moment between the trigger and the eating behavior.

C — CLARIFY

Name what just happened. Not what you felt — what occurred. Ask: What actually just happened? What story am I telling about it? • Separate the event from the interpretation • Name the distorted thought if present • Ask: is this fact or story?

O — OBSERVE

Scan the body without judgment. Notice where the emotion lives physically. Ask: Where do I feel this in my body right now? • Take one slow breath — in 4 counts, hold 2, out 4 • Scan from head to chest to stomach to hands • Name the sensation: tight, hot, heavy, hollow • Acknowledge: I feel this. It will pass.

P — PAUSE

Create a gap between the trigger and the action. The pause is where choice lives. Ask: Am I willing to do what it takes to stay aligned? • 4-second breathing: in 4, hold 2, out 4 — repeat 3 times • 5-4-3-2-1 grounding: 5 things you see, 4 you hear, 3 touch, 2 smell, 1 taste • Physical step away from the food or trigger • Set a 3-minute timer before any eating decision

E — EXECUTE

Take the next aligned action. Not the perfect action. The smallest step forward. Ask: What is the one aligned action I can take right now? • Use if-then planning: if I feel X, then I will do Y • Stack the new behavior onto an existing one • Return to the stage coach — there is no starting over, only continuing

THE FOUR FORCES — QUICK REFERENCE

C.O.P.E. works best when you can name which force is driving the urge. Use this reference to identify the force, then return to C.O.P.E. to navigate it.

WHAT'S HAPPENING
WHAT TO DO
A stressful day or difficult moment
Clarify what triggered it. Name the emotion. Pause with four slow breaths. Then take the one action you already decided on.
Late-night loneliness or boredom
Name it: this is loneliness, not hunger. Observe where it lives in your body. Reach out to someone, or journal for five minutes.
Food is sitting right in front of you
Remove it from the space. If you can't, put distance between yourself and it. What you can't see, you're less likely to reach for.
A craving for a specific memory food
Ask: am I hungry, or am I trying to return to a moment? If it's a memory, name the moment. That's what you're actually after.
You've already eaten something off-plan
The stage coach is still running. One off-plan choice doesn't end the day. Execute the next right thing.
Hunger that won't soften after eating
This may be a disease signal, not an emotional one. Walk — the pre-decided, already-practiced walk. Do not try to satisfy it with food.

The Four Forces That Drive Non-Hunger Eating Every eating event that is not driven by physiological hunger is driven by one or more of these four forces.

H — HABIT Eating triggered by environmental cues, routines, and automatic patterns — not hunger. Core question: What in my environment is triggering this behavior? Strategy: Identify the cue. Change the environment. Build a competing routine.

E — EMOTION Eating as a response to emotional states — stress, loneliness, boredom, anxiety, or celebration. Core question: What am I actually feeling right now that has nothing to do with hunger? Strategy: Use C.O.P.E. Name the emotion. Find a non-food way to meet the need.

A — ACCESS Eating because the food is present, convenient, and requires no decision to reach for. Core question: Would I have eaten this if it required effort to obtain? Strategy: Redesign the environment. Increase friction for foods that work against you.

T — TASTE Eating driven by memory, emotional association, and the sensory experience that a specific food produces. Core question: Am I eating this food, or am I trying to eat what it represents? Strategy: Trace the story behind the taste. Distinguish between memory- based taste and engineered craving.

THE BLISS POINT — THE FIFTH DIMENSION OF TASTE Engineered food is designed to operate outside of hunger. The bliss point creates a craving cycle that the H.E.A.T. Taste force alone does not fully explain. Recognition: If you cannot eat just one, if the food produces a pleasure surge followed by incomplete satisfaction, the craving returns stronger after eating. Response: Environmental design is the primary tool. The solution is not willpower in the moment of contact.

FREQUENTLY ASKED QUESTIONS

The questions in this section are the ones I have been asked most often. By patients, in clinical encounters. By Accelerators, in our community. By audiences. By family members of patients, in the doorway after the appointment is over.

I have organized them by category. Read what is relevant to you. Skip what is not.

Two important notes before we begin. First, the answers below are general educational responses, not medical advice for your specific situation. Every answer here should be brought to your healthcare provider for the conversation that fits your case. These responses are educational. Your healthcare provider knows your medical history, your medications, your laboratory values, and your circumstances in a way no book can. Use these answers to understand what is possible. Use your healthcare provider to understand what is right for you.

Second, on the question of medications. Several questions below address medication classes by their general category rather than by brand name. The drug landscape changes quickly. The principles below apply across the major medication classes used in diabetes care; your healthcare provider can speak to your specific medications and adjustments.

—

ABOUT YOUR DISEASE

1. What is the difference between type 2 diabetes and prediabetes?

The difference is one of degree, not kind. Both reflect the same underlying problem: the body's cells have become less responsive to insulin's signal, the pancreas is producing more insulin to compensate, and blood sugar is beginning to rise. Prediabetes means the rise has crossed a threshold that puts you at higher risk of full diabetes within a few years. Type 2 diabetes means the rise has crossed a higher threshold, and the consequences of untreated disease are now beginning to accumulate.

The framework in this book applies to both. Prediabetes is often the easier case to address, because the body has typically not yet experienced the long-term effects of years of elevated blood sugar. If you are reading this with prediabetes, you have a window many patients with full diabetes wish they had taken seriously when they had it.

2. If I do not have diabetes but my fasting glucose is creeping up, is the framework relevant to me?

Yes. A creeping fasting glucose is one of the body's earlier visible signals that insulin resistance may be developing. The framework in this book is built to address that root mechanism, regardless of whether you have crossed any specific diagnostic threshold. Discuss the trend with your healthcare provider, who can determine whether further evaluation is appropriate for your situation.

3. Can type 1 diabetes be reversed using this framework?

No. Type 1 diabetes is an autoimmune condition in which the immune system has destroyed the beta cells that produce insulin. People with type 1 diabetes will require insulin replacement for life, and any changes to insulin therapy must be made under the direct supervision of their endocrinologist. The metabolic principles taught in this book may improve overall health and protect against the cardiovascular and metabolic complications that can develop alongside type 1 disease, but the disease itself does not reverse. If you have type 1 diabetes, work with your endocrinologist to understand whether and how the principles here might serve as supportive practices alongside your insulin therapy. Do not adjust insulin without your healthcare provider's involvement.

4. Is type 2 diabetes really reversible, or will I always have it?

Type 2 diabetes is reversible for many patients. The American Diabetes Association, together with several other major diabetes organizations, published a consensus report defining diabetes remission: an A1C below 6.5 percent for at least three months without the use of glucose-lowering medications. That criterion exists because remission is now well-documented as a real clinical outcome.

Whether your specific diabetes is reversible depends on factors including how long you have had the disease, how much beta cell function remains, your genetics, and your individual circumstances. Many patients reach remission. Some reach what I would call a much better managed state, where their numbers are normal or near-normal but they remain on a low dose of one or two medications. Both outcomes are meaningful. Both represent significant improvement over the trajectory of unaddressed type 2 diabetes. Your healthcare provider is the right person to assess what outcome is most realistic for you.

5. What does it mean if my A1C is normal but my fasting blood sugar is high?

This pattern is more common than it sometimes seems. The A1C is a three-month average of your blood sugar; a normal A1C with elevated fasting glucose can suggest that your body is overcorrecting overnight or after meals, which can mask morning elevations. It can also be one of the earlier signals that insulin resistance is developing, even before the standard diagnostic criteria have been met.

If this is your pattern, bring it up with your healthcare provider. The framework in this book is designed for exactly this stage, when intervention is often most straightforward, but your healthcare provider is best positioned to determine whether further evaluation is warranted.

—

ABOUT MEDICATIONS

1. What if my doctor takes a different approach than this book describes?

This question deserves a careful answer, because most patients who ask it are working with a physician they trust and are simply trying to understand whether the work in this book complements their existing care.

The good news is that the lifestyle principles in this book are widely supported across the medical profession. Walking, strength training, balanced nutrition, sleep, stress management, and structured habits are recommendations that nearly every physician supports. The framework in this book organizes those principles into a structure designed for sustained application, but the foundations are not controversial.

Where physicians sometimes differ is on the question of how aggressively to pursue diabetes reversal as a treatment goal versus continued medication management. This is a clinical conversation, and reasonable physicians can land in different places based on their training, their experience, and their assessment of an individual patient. If your healthcare provider's approach differs from what you are reading here, that does not mean either of you is wrong. It means you have an opportunity to have a richer conversation.

A reasonable way to open that conversation is to share what you are doing, share what you are reading, and ask how to integrate the lifestyle work with the medical care you are already receiving. Most physicians appreciate engaged patients who are taking ownership of their health. Your healthcare provider knows your full picture in a way no book can.

If after that conversation you still feel your goals and your healthcare provider's approach are not aligned, it is reasonable to seek additional perspectives. Many patients benefit from working with both a primary care provider and a specialist in metabolic health. Taking ownership of your health is always appropriate.

2. What if I am on insulin? Can I still apply the principles in this book?

This is a question for your healthcare provider, and it must be answered in the context of strict medical supervision.

The general principle is that the lifestyle work in this book reduces the body's need for insulin over time. As that happens, insulin doses must be adjusted downward, or low blood sugar (hypoglycemia) becomes a real risk. That dose adjustment is a clinical decision that your healthcare provider makes, not one you make on your own.

If you are on insulin and want to begin applying the principles in this book, the right starting point is a conversation with your healthcare provider about how to proceed safely. Most physicians will support a graduated approach: increased blood sugar monitoring, gradual lifestyle changes, and stepwise medication adjustments based on the response. The work is possible. The work must be supervised.

3. What if I am taking metformin or other oral diabetes medications?

The general class of oral diabetes medications is well tolerated by most patients. As your numbers improve through lifestyle work, your healthcare provider may consider adjusting or discontinuing some of these medications. Some classes of oral medications carry a higher risk of low blood sugar than others, and the urgency of dose adjustment varies accordingly. Your healthcare provider knows which class you are on and what the appropriate adjustments would be.

Some patients choose, in conversation with their healthcare provider, to remain on a low dose of certain medications even after achieving normal blood sugar, because some of these medications have been associated with potential benefits beyond glucose control. That is a clinical conversation worth having with your healthcare provider.

4. What about the newer weight-loss and diabetes medications I keep hearing about?

You are likely referring to a class of medications known as GLP-1 receptor agonists, and a related class known as dual GLP-1 and GIP agonists. These medications have transformed the conversation about weight and metabolic disease. They produce significant weight loss and meaningful improvements in blood sugar in most patients who take them. Whether any of these medications are appropriate for you is a conversation for your healthcare provider.

What I can offer here is a perspective on how these medications relate to the framework in this book. These medications work primarily by reducing appetite and slowing gastric emptying, which makes it easier to eat less. They do not, on their own, teach the patterns, identity, and design that produce sustainable health independent of the medication. Patients who lose weight on these medications and stop taking them, without doing the underlying work, often regain most of the weight within a year.

If you and your healthcare provider decide a medication in this category is appropriate for you, the framework in this book is exactly the work I would recommend doing alongside it. Use the time and capacity the medication gives you to build the patterns that will sustain the results when the medication is eventually tapered. The medication can be a powerful tool. It is not a substitute for the work this book teaches.

5. What if I have other conditions besides diabetes? High blood pressure, high cholesterol, heart disease, kidney disease?

The conditions you list often travel alongside type 2 diabetes, because they share the same metabolic root: insulin resistance and the inflammatory state that comes with it. The framework in this book addresses the root, which means it tends to support improvement in these conditions in parallel.

Improvement in these conditions often means that your medications may need adjustment over time. As blood pressure normalizes, blood pressure medications may be reconsidered. As lipid profiles improve, statin therapy may be revisited. As kidney function stabilizes, your healthcare provider may revisit your medication choices.

All of this happens in conversation with your healthcare provider, not on your own. The point is that the work you are doing on diabetes is also working on the broader picture of your metabolic health. The medication adjustments may follow your progress, and your healthcare provider is the one who guides those adjustments.

—

ABOUT IMPLEMENTATION

1. How long will it take to see results?

Most patients I have worked with see meaningful improvement in blood sugar within two to four weeks of consistently applying the framework. Energy often improves within the same window. Weight loss is more variable; some patients see it quickly, others take longer.

A1C, because it is a three-month average, takes three months to fully reflect what your blood sugar has been doing. Do not be discouraged if your A1C drops less dramatically than your daily numbers in the first month. The A1C will catch up.

Patients who achieve remission typically do so within six to twelve months of consistently applying the framework, though the timeline varies considerably. Your specific timeline depends on factors your healthcare provider can help you assess: how long you have had the disease, how completely you can apply the framework, and the support around you.

2. What if I plateau?

Plateaus are a normal part of the process and almost always have a specific cause. The most common causes I see in my practice are these: sleep has degraded without you noticing; stress has increased; the food has crept back toward old patterns through a series of small concessions you have not added up; strength training has dropped off; the walk after dinner has become a walk after dinner three days a week.

When you plateau, the move is rarely to increase the intensity of what you have been doing. The move is to audit. Look at the seven pillars and find the one or two that have slipped. Restore them. The plateau usually breaks within a few weeks of returning to the basics. If it does not, bring it up with your healthcare provider — there may be a clinical factor worth investigating.

3. What if I get off track?

You will, at some point. Most patients do.

The work is not about never getting off track. The work is about what happens after you do.

The single most useful behavior I see in patients who succeed long term is the ability to return to the framework quickly after a deviation, without spending two weeks in self-recrimination. They eat a meal that does not align with the framework. The next meal, they return to the framework. They miss two days of walks. The third day, they walk. They have a bad week. The next week, they begin again.

Patients who struggle most are the ones who treat a single bad meal as evidence that the whole effort has failed, and then spend three weeks proving themselves right. The framework is forgiving of mistakes. It is the abandonment that creates the problem.

4. How do I afford this if I do not have the budget for monitors and special foods?

The framework does not require any specific tools or special foods. It requires the application of principles. Walking after meals is free. Strength training with body weight is free. Sleeping in a cool, dark room is free. Eating real food at the perimeter of the grocery store is often less expensive than eating processed food in the interior aisles, because the unit cost of whole food per gram of nutrition is lower.

The most expensive parts of this work are tools that make the work easier and tools that make invisible patterns visible: continuous glucose monitors, sleep trackers, body composition scales. These tools are useful but not required. Many patients do this work successfully without any of them. If your budget is constrained, focus on the principles. Add tools as you can.

5. Do I need to follow a specific diet?

The framework in this book is not a specific diet. It is an approach to eating that emphasizes protein and healthy fats, real and minimally processed foods, controlled carbohydrates, and meal timing that supports insulin reduction. Within those principles, several specific approaches can work — Mediterranean, low-carbohydrate, ketogenic, and whole-food plant-forward approaches each have evidence supporting their use in metabolic health.

What I have observed in clinical practice is that approaches relying heavily on processed substitutes, requiring obsessive calorie counting, or ignoring the role of sleep, stress, movement, and structure tend to be harder to sustain. The diet alone is not the framework. The diet is one part of a larger design. Discuss the specifics of how to apply this with your healthcare provider or with a registered dietitian who is familiar with metabolic health.

6. What if I live with a partner or family who is not doing this with me?

Read Chapter Eleven. The relational dimension is real, and the chapter addresses it directly. The two-sentence exercise from Chapter Eleven is the most concrete intervention I can offer here, and many patients who practice it find that the household becomes more supportive over time.

In the meantime, focus on what you can control. Your meals. Your walks. Your sleep. Your work. The household will often adapt as your results become visible.

—

ABOUT THE FRAMEWORK

1. What if H.E.A.T. does not seem to apply to me?

H.E.A.T. is a model for the four most common drivers of non-hunger eating. Not every driver is equally present in every patient. Some patients are heavily driven by Habit and barely affected by Emotion. Some are the reverse. Some are primarily Access. Some are primarily Taste.

If one of the four does not seem to apply to you, work on the ones that do. The model is a diagnostic tool for understanding what is driving you, not a checklist of behaviors you have to address in some specific order.

2. What if C.O.P.E. does not work in the moment?

C.O.P.E. requires practice. The first time you try it in the middle of a craving, it may feel slow and clumsy, and the craving may win. The second time, slightly less. By the tenth or twentieth time, it tends to begin interrupting the automatic behavior reliably.

If C.O.P.E. is not working for you after several attempts, the most common reason I see is that the cravings being addressed are not actually emotional. Some cravings are physiological: blood sugar has dropped, sleep has been poor, protein intake has been low. C.O.P.E. is designed for the emotional cravings. The physiological signals call for a different response — eat, sleep, stabilize. If you are unsure which kind of craving you are experiencing, that is also a useful conversation to have with your healthcare provider.

3. What about the seven pillars? Do I have to apply all seven at once?

No, and I would not recommend it. Most patients who try to do everything in week one tend to burn out by week three. Pick two pillars that fit your current life. Build them as habits over a month. Add a third. Then a fourth. The full structure of all seven pillars is the destination, not the starting point.

The order in which you build them matters less than the consistency with which you build them. Some patients begin with walking and food. Some begin with sleep and stress. Some begin with strength and structure. The right starting point is the one you will actually do.

4. What if I have read every diabetes book and tried everything and nothing has worked?

This experience is more common than it should be, and it is often the result of approaches that address only one or two of the variables that drive the disease. The framework in this book is built to address the broader picture: the metabolic, the behavioral, the emotional, the relational, and the structural. Patients who have not had success with single-variable approaches sometimes find that a more integrated approach produces different results.

If you have applied the work in this book completely and consistently for six months and seen no meaningful improvement in your numbers, that is rare but it does happen. In those cases, there is often a hidden variable: a thyroid issue, a cortisol disorder, a sleep apnea diagnosis that has not been made, a medication interaction, a genetic factor that requires a more specialized approach. The right next step is a thorough metabolic workup with your healthcare provider, who may refer you to an endocrinologist or another specialist who can look at the full picture.

—

A FINAL NOTE

If your question is not in this list, it is not because it does not matter. It is because there are more questions than fit in this section. Bring the questions you have to your healthcare provider, to your community, and to the broader resources listed elsewhere in this book.

The framework is meant to be applied, not memorized. Read what you need. Act on what is in front of you. Bring the rest to the people in your life who are positioned to help you act on it well.

RECOMMENDED LABS

The standard panel ordered at most diabetes follow-up appointments is a perfectly reasonable set of tests. It typically includes A1C, a basic metabolic panel, and a lipid panel, and it answers the questions that most diabetes care needs answered. Your healthcare provider knows your history, has been trained extensively in this work, and is the right person to determine what tests are appropriate for you.

This section is not meant to replace that judgment. It is meant to give you a vocabulary so that the conversation in your appointment can go further than it sometimes has time to go. The list below is a set of tests that I commonly use with my own patients walking through this framework. Bring it to your next appointment as a list of labs to discuss with your healthcare provider. Some of these will already be part of your regular workup. Some your healthcare provider may add based on your specific situation. Some your healthcare provider may reasonably decline as not necessary for your case. All of those outcomes are appropriate.

A note on insurance. Most of these tests are covered by standard insurance for patients with a diabetes diagnosis or a metabolic syndrome workup. A few may require a specific request or be paid out of pocket. Costs vary; ask your healthcare provider's office or your laboratory.

A reminder. The values listed below are general targets based on current research and clinical practice. They are not a substitute for the interpretation of a physician who knows your full medical history. Ranges for some tests are updated periodically as guidelines evolve. If a value here differs from what your healthcare provider is using, follow your healthcare provider's guidance — the clinical context always takes precedence. Bring your results to your healthcare provider. Use the framework here to ask better questions. Do not adjust medications based on lab values without your healthcare provider's involvement.

—

THE CORE PANEL

These are the tests that show whether your blood sugar and insulin response are healthy, whether the disease is moving in the direction of remission, and whether the work you are doing is producing measurable change. Most of these are routinely ordered as part of standard diabetes follow-up.

Hemoglobin A1C

What it measures. The percentage of hemoglobin in your blood that has glucose attached to it. Because red blood cells live for about three months, the A1C is effectively a three-month average of your blood sugar.

What the targets look like. Below 5.7 percent is non-diabetic. 5.7 to 6.4 percent is prediabetes. 6.5 percent and above indicates diabetes. The American Diabetes Association definition of remission is an A1C below 6.5 percent for at least three months without glucose-lowering medication.

What an out-of-range value tells you. An elevated A1C reflects that your blood sugar has been running higher than it should over the past three months. It does not tell you when, how often, or under what conditions. For that more granular picture, your healthcare provider may suggest a continuous glucose monitor or fingerstick monitoring at specific times of day.

How often it is typically tested. Every three months while actively reversing. Every six months once you have reached remission and are stable.

Fasting glucose

What it measures. Your blood sugar after at least eight hours without food, typically tested first thing in the morning before breakfast.

What the targets look like. 70 to 99 mg/dL is normal. 100 to 125 mg/dL is prediabetes. 126 mg/dL and above on two separate occasions is diabetes.

What an out-of-range value tells you. An elevated fasting glucose despite a normal A1C can suggest that your body is running high overnight or in the morning, even if your daytime numbers are reasonable. This is sometimes an early sign of insulin resistance worth discussing with your healthcare provider.

How often it is typically tested. Anytime you have other labs drawn. The fasting glucose comes as part of most metabolic panels.

Fasting insulin

What it measures. Your blood insulin level after at least eight hours without food.

What the targets look like. Below 10 μIU/mL. Optimally, below 6 to 8.

What an out-of-range value tells you. A fasting insulin in the teens or twenties suggests that the pancreas is working harder than usual to keep your blood sugar in the normal range. Your A1C may still be normal, your fasting glucose may still be normal, but the body is laboring against insulin resistance underneath. Some physicians order this routinely; others order it when there is reason to look for early insulin resistance. Worth asking about if it is not already part of your workup.

How often it is typically tested. Every six months at minimum, when ordered.

Comprehensive metabolic panel

What it measures. A panel of fourteen tests that includes glucose, kidney function (creatinine, BUN, and eGFR), liver function (AST, ALT, alkaline phosphatase, bilirubin), electrolytes (sodium, potassium, chloride, CO_2, calcium), and total protein.

What out-of-range values tell you. Elevated liver enzymes (AST and ALT) often signal fatty liver disease, which is closely tied to insulin resistance. Elevated creatinine, or a low eGFR (estimated glomerular filtration rate, which most labs calculate automatically from your creatinine), signals reduced kidney function — which can develop after years of poorly controlled blood sugar. eGFR is worth looking at directly on your report; values above 90 are normal, 60 to 89 are mildly reduced, and anything below 60 deserves a conversation. Electrolyte abnormalities can develop with significant dietary changes or with certain medications.

How often it is typically tested. At least annually at minimum. More often if any individual value has been abnormal.

GGT (gamma-glutamyl transferase)

What it measures. A liver enzyme that often becomes elevated before the more familiar AST and ALT enzymes show change. GGT is sometimes referred to as one of the earliest detectable signs of fatty liver disease.

What the targets look like. Reference ranges vary by laboratory and by sex, typically below 40 U/L for women and below 50 U/L for men.

What an out-of-range value tells you. Elevated GGT can signal early fatty liver disease, alcohol-related liver stress, or biliary tract issues. In the context of metabolic disease specifically, an elevated GGT alongside other signs of insulin resistance is one of the earlier warning signs that the liver is being affected. Lifestyle changes that reverse insulin resistance often produce measurable improvement in GGT before changes show in AST or ALT. Sometimes ordered routinely as part of an extended liver panel; sometimes added when there is a specific reason to look at liver function more closely. Worth asking about if it is not already on your panel.

How often it is typically tested. Annually when included in the workup.

Urine microalbumin-to-creatinine ratio

What it measures. The amount of a small protein called albumin that leaks from your blood into your urine, divided by the amount of creatinine. Tested from a simple urine sample. Normal kidneys do not allow albumin to pass into the urine; even small amounts of albumin (microalbumin) can be one of the earliest signs of kidney stress.

What the targets look like. Below 30 mg/g is normal. 30 to 300 mg/g is moderately increased albumin (sometimes called microalbuminuria). Above 300 mg/g is severely increased.

What an out-of-range value tells you. An elevated microalbumin-to-creatinine ratio is one of the earliest signals that diabetes may be affecting kidney function. Catching it early opens the door to interventions that can slow or reverse the progression. The good news for patients walking through the framework in this book: improvements in blood sugar and blood pressure often produce measurable improvements in this ratio over time.

How often it is typically tested. At least annually for patients with type 2 diabetes. More often if previous values have been elevated.

C-peptide

What it measures. A protein released by the pancreas in equal proportion to insulin every time insulin is produced. Because insulin is cleared rapidly from the blood while C-peptide is cleared more slowly, measuring C-peptide gives a more stable picture of how much insulin your pancreas is actually making.

What the targets look like. Reference ranges vary by laboratory. The interpretation matters more than the absolute number.

What an out-of-range value tells you. C-peptide helps answer a question that fasting insulin alone cannot fully answer: how much insulin-producing capacity does the pancreas have left? A low C-peptide in someone with diabetes suggests that beta cell function has declined significantly. A normal or elevated C-peptide in someone with diabetes suggests that the pancreas is still producing insulin, and that insulin resistance is the dominant problem rather than insulin deficiency. This distinction can meaningfully influence treatment decisions, including whether certain medications are appropriate. Often ordered when there is a question about how much beta cell function remains.

How often it is typically tested. As clinically indicated, rather than routinely.

Complete blood count

What it measures. A panel of tests on the cells in your blood. Includes red blood cell count, white blood cell count, platelets, hemoglobin, and hematocrit.

What out-of-range values tell you. Anemia, infection, inflammatory states, and bleeding disorders all show up on this panel. While not specific to diabetes, the CBC catches issues that can complicate diabetes management.

How often it is typically tested. At least annually.

—

THE CARDIOVASCULAR AND LIPID PANEL

Cardiovascular disease is the leading cause of death in patients with type 2 diabetes. Current guidelines from the American College of Cardiology and the American Heart Association have updated several recommendations relevant to patients with diabetes. The tests below reflect current guidance and provide the most complete picture available of cardiovascular risk and progress.

Lipid panel (full)

What it measures. Total cholesterol, LDL cholesterol, HDL cholesterol, triglycerides.

What the targets look like. The targets that matter most for metabolic health are triglycerides below 100 mg/dL (the standard clinical cutoff is below 150 mg/dL; below 100 is the metabolic optimization target used here) and HDL above 60 mg/dL. Total cholesterol and LDL targets vary based on your overall cardiovascular risk and the most current guidelines, and are best discussed with your healthcare provider.

What out-of-range values tell you. Elevated triglycerides are one of the more reliable signs of insulin resistance. Low HDL is the second. The pattern of high triglycerides plus low HDL is often more telling for metabolic health than the total cholesterol or LDL number, both of which can be elevated for reasons unrelated to insulin resistance.

How often it is typically tested. Every six to twelve months while actively reversing.

Triglyceride-to-HDL ratio

What it measures. A simple division: triglycerides divided by HDL.

What the targets look like. Below 2.0 is optimal. 2.0 to 3.0 is borderline. Above 3.0 strongly suggests insulin resistance.

What an out-of-range value tells you. This single ratio is, in much of the metabolic health literature, considered a useful surrogate marker for insulin resistance available from a standard lipid panel. Many laboratories calculate it automatically; if yours does not, the ratio is easy to calculate from your existing lipid results.

How often it is typically tested. Every time you have a lipid panel drawn.

Non-HDL cholesterol

What it measures. Your total cholesterol minus your HDL cholesterol. This number captures all of the cholesterol in your blood that is not the protective HDL fraction.

What the targets look like. Below 130 mg/dL for general targets. Lower targets apply for patients with diabetes or established cardiovascular disease, per current guidelines.

What an out-of-range value tells you. Non-HDL cholesterol is now formally recommended in current guidelines as a treatment target alongside LDL, particularly in patients with diabetes. Many laboratories now report this value automatically. If yours does not, it is easy to calculate.

How often it is typically tested. Every six to twelve months.

Lipoprotein(a), or Lp(a)

What it measures. Lp(a) is a type of LDL particle attached to a specific protein. Levels are largely determined by genetics and remain relatively stable over a lifetime.

What the targets look like. Below 30 mg/dL or below 75 nmol/L is generally desirable. Levels of 50 mg/dL or 125 nmol/L and above are associated with increased cardiovascular risk. Levels above 250 nmol/L are associated with substantially increased risk.

What an out-of-range value tells you. Elevated Lp(a) is a genetically determined risk factor that lifestyle changes do not significantly affect. Current ACC/AHA guidelines now recommend measuring Lp(a) at least once in adulthood for every adult, in part because it identifies people who may need more aggressive management of other risk factors. This is a one-time test for most patients. Worth discussing with your healthcare provider if it has never been measured.

How often it is typically tested. Once in adulthood is generally sufficient.

ApoB (Apolipoprotein B)

What it measures. The protein attached to every atherogenic lipoprotein particle in your blood. Each LDL, VLDL, and Lp(a) particle carries one ApoB, so the ApoB count is effectively a count of the particles in your blood that can deposit cholesterol in your arteries.

What the targets look like. Below 90 mg/dL for general targets. Below 80 mg/dL or lower for patients with diabetes or established cardiovascular disease, depending on overall risk profile.

What an out-of-range value tells you. Current ACC/AHA Dyslipidemia guidelines formally recommend ApoB measurement, particularly in patients with diabetes, hypertriglyceridemia, or low LDL cholesterol, because standard

LDL measurements can underestimate true risk in these populations. Sometimes ordered routinely, sometimes ordered when LDL and non-HDL targets have been met but residual risk is suspected. Worth a conversation with your healthcare provider about whether it is appropriate for your case.

How often it is typically tested. Annually when included in the workup.

hsCRP (high-sensitivity C-reactive protein)

What it measures. Inflammation in the body, at a level of sensitivity high enough to detect the chronic low-grade inflammation associated with metabolic disease.

What the targets look like. Below 1.0 mg/L is optimal. 1.0 to 3.0 is moderate cardiovascular risk. Above 3.0 indicates significant inflammation.

What an out-of-range value tells you. Chronic inflammation links insulin resistance, cardiovascular disease, and the long-term complications of diabetes. An elevated hsCRP that is not explained by an acute illness or injury suggests an inflammatory state worth discussing with your healthcare provider. One of the more sensitive markers for tracking improvement as you implement lifestyle changes.

How often it is typically tested. Every six months while actively reversing, when ordered.

—

THE HORMONE AND METABOLIC PANEL

Insulin is the central hormone in the metabolic story this book tells, but it is not the only hormone that affects metabolic health. The tests below cover the hormones most likely to interact with the disease and are commonly ordered when there is reason to look beyond the standard panel.

TSH (Thyroid Stimulating Hormone)

What it measures. The hormone the pituitary gland releases to tell the thyroid gland to produce thyroid hormone.

What the targets look like. The standard reference range runs from approximately 0.4 to 4.5 mIU/L.

What an out-of-range value tells you. An elevated TSH suggests an underactive thyroid (hypothyroidism), which slows metabolism, contributes to weight gain, and complicates diabetes management. A suppressed TSH suggests an overactive thyroid. Both are worth evaluating with your healthcare provider.

Free T3 and Free T4

What they measure. The active thyroid hormones circulating in your blood, distinct from the bound forms that are inactive.

What the targets look like. Most laboratories provide reference ranges. Some clinicians prefer Free T3 in the upper portion of the reference range and Free T4 in the middle of the reference range for optimal metabolic function.

What out-of-range values tell you. TSH alone can be normal while Free T3 and Free T4 are sub-optimal, particularly in patients with subclinical thyroid dysfunction. Adding Free T3 and Free T4 gives a more complete thyroid picture. Often added when initial TSH results raise questions.

Vitamin D (25-hydroxyvitamin D)

What it measures. Your stored vitamin D level, the most reliable measure of overall vitamin D status.

What the targets look like. Standard clinical sufficiency is above 30 ng/mL; 50 to 80 ng/mL reflects metabolic health optimization targets that some clinicians prefer.

What an out-of-range value tells you. Vitamin D deficiency is associated with insulin resistance and a long list of other conditions. Restoring vitamin D to the optimal range, through some combination of sun exposure, dietary sources, and supplementation, is one of the simpler interventions available. Discuss supplementation with your healthcare provider.

Uric acid

What it measures. The level of uric acid in your blood. Uric acid is a byproduct of fructose metabolism and certain other dietary patterns.

What the targets look like. Below 5.5 mg/dL.

What an out-of-range value tells you. Elevated uric acid is associated with insulin resistance, fatty liver disease, hypertension, and gout. Reducing dietary fructose, particularly from sweetened beverages and ultra-processed foods, often lowers uric acid significantly.

Magnesium

What it measures. The level of magnesium in your blood. Magnesium is a cofactor in more than three hundred enzymatic reactions, including those that govern insulin signaling.

What the targets look like. Within the laboratory's reference range, ideally in the upper half.

What an out-of-range value tells you. Low magnesium is associated with insulin resistance and is common in patients with type 2 diabetes. Worth discussing with your healthcare provider whether dietary changes or supplementation are appropriate for you.

—

A LIST TO BRING TO YOUR APPOINTMENT

If your next appointment is a regular diabetes follow-up, you do not need to ask for any of these. Your healthcare provider already orders most of them, and the conversation tends to flow naturally. If you would like to ask about adding tests beyond the standard panel, the list below is a reasonable starting point for that conversation.

Tests commonly part of routine diabetes follow-up:

* Hemoglobin A1C

* Fasting glucose

* Comprehensive metabolic panel

* Complete blood count

* Lipid panel

* Urine microalbumin-to-creatinine ratio (annually)

Tests sometimes ordered based on individual circumstances, worth discussing if not already part of your workup:

* Fasting insulin

* C-peptide

* GGT (gamma-glutamyl transferase)

* Lp(a) (one-time measurement per current guidelines)

* ApoB

* hsCRP

* TSH (with Free T3 and Free T4 if there is reason to look further)

* 25-hydroxyvitamin D

* Uric acid

* Magnesium

A simple way to open the conversation: *"I have been reading about some additional tests that can be useful for tracking metabolic health. I would love to know your thoughts on whether any of these are appropriate for my situation."* Your healthcare provider will tell you which fit your case and which do not. Either answer is a good answer.

If your healthcare provider declines particular tests as not standard for your case, that is a clinically reasonable decision. Many of the tests in the second list are situational, and your healthcare provider knows your full picture. You can always ask the reasoning behind the decision and learn from it.

—

A FINAL NOTE ON LABS

The labs are not the work. The labs are the feedback that tells you whether the work is working.

Some patients become anxious about their numbers and check them too often. Others avoid checking because they are afraid of what they will find. Both are versions of the same problem: a relationship with the numbers that is more emotional than analytical.

The right relationship with your labs is the one you would have with any other measurement of progress. Check at reasonable intervals. Look at the trends over time, not the snapshot. Bring the results to your healthcare provider and discuss them together. Use the data to refine what you are doing.

The numbers are telling you a story. The framework in this book is teaching you how to read it.

RESOURCES

The following is a guide to the categories of resources that extend the work this book introduces. Specific tools and platforms in each category change quickly. Rather than name them here and have them go out of date, I have organized this section around the kind of tool you should look for, what it should do, and what to ask before you commit to using it.

A note before you begin. Different readers will need different combinations of these resources. Some of you will use almost everything in this section. Some of you will use almost nothing in it and walk through the exit anyway. There is no required combination. What matters is that the resources you do choose serve the work, not that you assemble all of them.

—

MONITORING YOUR BODY

Continuous glucose monitors

A continuous glucose monitor is a small sensor worn on the back of the upper arm that measures glucose levels in real time. For most patients walking through this framework, a CGM transforms the experience of managing blood sugar from guesswork to feedback. You see what your body is doing in response to what you eat, how you sleep, and how you move. The data closes the gap between intention and observation.

Two categories of CGM are now available. The traditional category requires a prescription and is usually covered by insurance for patients with a diabetes diagnosis. A newer category is available over the counter without a prescription, designed for adults who want to monitor their glucose for general metabolic health. The over-the-counter options are paid out of pocket. Costs vary; expect to pay for the convenience.

Blood glucose meters

For patients who do not need continuous monitoring or who want a backup to a CGM, a standard at-home glucose meter remains useful. Look for one with reliable strip availability and a strong accuracy reputation. Test strips are the recurring cost; verify pricing before committing to a particular device.

If you are doing therapeutic carbohydrate restriction or extended fasting and want to verify ketone production, dual-purpose meters that measure both glucose and blood ketones from the same device are widely available. These are useful but not essential for most patients.

Body composition

A standard bathroom scale is sufficient for most patients. For those who want more detail, body composition scales that estimate body fat percentage, visceral fat, and lean mass are widely available at reasonable prices.

A reminder. Weight is one signal among many. Body composition matters more than the number on the scale. Waist circumference matters more than weight alone. Strength and energy matter more than either. Do not let the scale become the measurement that decides whether you are succeeding.

—

FOOD AND COOKING

Where to find recipes that align with this framework

Look for recipe sources that emphasize whole foods, that lead with protein and healthy fats, that treat carbohydrates as a smaller part of the plate rather than the center of it, and that do not depend on processed substitutes for the foods they are replacing. Subscription recipe sites focused on low-carbohydrate, real-food cooking are widely available and worth the modest cost during the months when you are rebuilding your kitchen habits.

Avoid recipe sources that rely heavily on artificial sweeteners, processed protein bars, and ultra-processed substitutes for natural foods. The goal is not to recreate the taste profile of the diet that was making you sick. The goal is to retrain your taste toward foods that nourish.

Tools that lower the friction of cooking at home

A pressure cooker or multi-function electric cooker. Speeds preparation of meats, beans, soups, and stews, removing one of the most common excuses for not cooking at home.

A sharp chef's knife and a stable cutting board. The right tools are surprisingly often the actual difference between cooking and not cooking. A sharp knife and a stable cutting surface remove the friction that keeps people from preparing fresh food.

A digital food scale. Useful in the early weeks of changing how you eat, when portion sizes have not yet recalibrated. After three or four months, most people no longer need it.

Meal planning

The most effective meal planning is not complex. It requires one decision made in advance: what protein and healthy fat anchor each meal. Everything else builds around that combination. Spend fifteen minutes at the start of each week identifying your protein and fat sources for the next seven days. The rest of the meal assembles itself.

Eating away from home

Eating away from home does not require a separate strategy. It requires the same framework applied to a different environment. Lead with protein and healthy fat. Ask how things are prepared. Request substitutions without apology. Most restaurants will accommodate a simple request. The meal does not have to be perfect. It has to be aligned.

Batch cooking and food preparation

Removing friction from good food is one of the highest-leverage changes you can make. Cook protein and prepare healthy fat sources in large batches once or twice a week. Pre-cut vegetables. Pre-portion nuts and other snacks. The goal is to make the aligned choice the easy choice — so that when the H.E.A.T. Access force activates, what is within reach is what serves you.

A note on grocery shopping

The single most consequential change you can make in your relationship with food is shifting where you shop. Try, for one month, doing eighty percent of your grocery shopping at the perimeter of the store and at a local farmer's market when possible. The perimeter is where the produce, the meats, the eggs, and the dairy live. The interior aisles are where most of the engineered hyperpalatable products live. The shopping route changes the food. The food changes the body.

—

MOVEMENT AND STRENGTH

You do not need a gym membership to follow this framework. You do need to move, and you do need to load your muscles with resistance regularly. Both can be done at home with minimal equipment.

For walking and daily movement

A pedometer or smartwatch that tracks daily step count. The point is not the device. The point is making your daily movement visible to yourself. Most patients I see have no idea how few steps they actually take in a typical day until they begin tracking.

For patients who can no longer easily increase their walking time, a weighted vest can intensify the same daily walk without adding minutes. Start light. Increase slowly.

For strength training at home

A pair of adjustable dumbbells. Replaces an entire rack of fixed weights and takes up far less space. Available at most sporting goods retailers.

A simple bench. A flat or slightly inclinable bench, available at most sporting goods retailers, allows you to perform the majority of upper-body strength exercises at home.

A doorway pull-up bar. Inexpensive, easily installed, and adds an entire category of strength work that is otherwise difficult to do at home.

How to find a program

Look for a beginner strength training program that emphasizes the major compound movements: squat, deadlift, press, row, and pull-up variations. Programs that focus on these movements train the whole body efficiently and build the kind of functional strength that supports the metabolic work you are doing in parallel.

If you are a woman in midlife, look specifically for programs designed around the metabolic and hormonal shifts that occur during perimenopause and menopause. These programs are increasingly available and address considerations that more general programs miss.

A note on starting

If you have been sedentary for years, do not start with intensity. Start with the smallest movement you can sustain. Two minutes of walking after each meal. Five push-ups against the wall when you wake up. A single set of squats while waiting for the coffee to brew. The intensity increases on its own once the habit is established. The habit will not establish itself if you start too hard and quit by the end of the second week.

—

REST AND RECOVERY

Sleep tracking

A wearable sleep tracker is useful for the same reason a CGM is useful. It makes invisible patterns visible. Look for a device that tracks sleep stages, heart rate variability, and recovery metrics.

Ring-worn and wrist-worn devices are both available at a range of price points. Subscription costs vary; verify before committing.

For improving sleep environment

A blackout curtain or sleep mask. Light suppression in the bedroom is consistently underrated as a metabolic intervention. Even small amounts of ambient light during sleep have been shown to disrupt glucose regulation the next day.

A bedroom thermostat set to sixty-five to sixty-eight degrees Fahrenheit. Sleep quality improves measurably in cooler bedrooms.

Removal of screens from the bedroom. The single change most patients resist and most patients benefit from when they finally make it. Read on paper. Charge the phone in another room.

For stress and recovery

Guided meditation apps are widely available. Look for one with a structured beginner program if you have never meditated, or with a deep library of unguided sessions if you are returning to a practice you have done before.

A simple breathwork practice you can do without an app: four seconds in, four seconds hold, six seconds out. Repeat for five cycles, twice a day. The practice trains the parasympathetic nervous system to engage on demand, which is precisely what is required to lower cortisol and improve insulin sensitivity over time.

—

COMMUNITY AND CONTINUED LEARNING

The Woode Life Design platform at dwainwoode.com is the home of the framework. The site includes the WLD Weekly Brief, video content, and free resources for readers.

For tools, resources, and continued learning connected to this book, visit thediabetesexit.com.

A note on what you choose to consume

Your information environment shapes your beliefs about what is possible. If the voices in your ears every day are telling you that diabetes is a life sentence and the best you can do is manage it, your beliefs will reflect that. If the voices in your ears are telling you that the disease is reversible, that the body is responsive to change, and that the framework you are learning has worked for thousands of people before you, your beliefs will reflect that. Choose carefully. Listen to the voices that match the future you are trying to build.

—

FOR THE PEOPLE AROUND YOU

Chapter Eleven addresses the relational dimension of this work directly. The following supports the people who are walking this with you.

For spouses, partners, and family members

Read Chapter Eleven together. Then read it again, in opposite directions: the partner reads the section addressed to the patient, and the patient reads the section addressed to the partner. The exercise is uncomfortable. The exercise is also exactly the work.

The two-sentence exercise from Chapter Eleven is meant to be practiced. Practice it once a week for a month. The relationship will change.

> **Person supporting:** *I know that managing diabetes is difficult.*
>
> **Person with diabetes:** *Thank you for caring. I give you permission to speak into my life.*

For adult children of a parent with diabetes

You did not cause your parent's disease, and you cannot manage it for them. Your job is to love them well. Your job is also to take seriously what their disease is teaching you about your own metabolic future. Both are true at the same time.

For employers and colleagues

A patient managing diabetes well does not need accommodations as much as they need understanding. The fifteen-minute walk after lunch, the absence at a 2 p.m. meeting once a quarter for an endocrinology appointment, the protein-forward food at the catered lunch, none of these are special requests. They are the daily infrastructure of someone treating their disease seriously. Your support of those small allowances is part of why they are succeeding.

For pastors and faith communities

If someone in your congregation is doing this work, what they need from you is not a sermon about discipline. What they need is the same thing your community is built to offer: presence, prayer, accountability, and the long view. The disease is not a moral failing. The reversal is not a moral victory. It is a body responding to design, and the support of a community walking with the person doing the work.

—

A FINAL NOTE ON RESOURCES

A book is a starting point, not an ending point. The framework in these pages is the architecture; the resources you choose are the materials with which you will build the house. There is no single correct combination.

What matters is that you build something. What matters is that the building, whatever shape it takes, is consistent with the design taught in these pages.

The exit is real. The materials to walk through it are within reach. The work begins the moment you decide it is time.

A PATIENT'S VOCABULARY

The terms in this section are the language of the disease. Some of them appear throughout this book. Others you will encounter on your lab reports, in conversation with your healthcare provider, and in your further reading. All of them are defined here at the patient level — written in plain language, organized alphabetically. The framework terms specific to the Woode Life Design framework appear here alongside the clinical terms, marked with the symbol * after the entry name.

—

A1C (HEMOGLOBIN A1C, HbA1c)

A blood test that measures the percentage of hemoglobin in your red blood cells that has glucose attached to it. Because red blood cells live for about three months, the A1C is effectively a three-month average of your blood sugar. Below 5.7 percent is non-diabetic; 5.7 to 6.4 is prediabetes; 6.5 and above is diabetes.

ACCELERATORS *

Members of the Woode Life Design community who are actively applying this framework. The term reflects the principle that the work is not waiting for permission, not waiting for the right time, not waiting for someone else to decide it is possible. Accelerators are people who chose to begin.

ANCHORS *

The structures, identities, and beliefs that hold a person steady when conditions are unstable. Anchors are what does not move when everything else does. In the context of this framework, anchors include your reasons, your relationships, and your core practices.

APOB (APOLIPOPROTEIN B)

A protein attached to every atherogenic lipoprotein particle in your blood. Each LDL, VLDL, and IDL particle has exactly one

ApoB on it, so an ApoB count is effectively a count of the cholesterol particles in your blood that can deposit cholesterol in your arteries. Increasingly recognized as one of the most accurate markers of cardiovascular risk available.

BETA CELL

The cell in your pancreas that produces insulin. Beta cells respond to rising blood sugar by releasing insulin, which signals the body to absorb glucose from the blood. Over many years of high insulin demand, beta cells can become exhausted and produce less insulin. The decline of beta cell function is one of the major drivers of progressive type 2 diabetes.

C.O.P.E. *

A real-time framework for the moments that have historically undone you. The four steps are Clarify (name what is happening), Observe (notice the body and the urge without judgment), Pause (insert space between the trigger and the action), and Execute (take the chosen action rather than the automatic one). C.O.P.E. operates in the gap between what you feel and what you do.

CARDIOVASCULAR DISEASE

Disease of the heart and blood vessels. The leading cause of death in patients with type 2 diabetes. The risk of cardiovascular disease is significantly elevated in patients with insulin resistance, regardless of whether the patient has crossed the diagnostic threshold for diabetes.

CGM

See Continuous Glucose Monitor.

CONTINUOUS GLUCOSE MONITOR

A small wearable device that measures glucose levels in real time. Readings update every few minutes. Allows patients to see directly how their blood sugar responds to food, sleep, stress, and movement. Available both over the counter and by prescription.

CORTISOL

The body's primary stress hormone. Released during physical or psychological stress to mobilize energy. Chronic elevation of cortisol contributes to insulin resistance, abdominal weight gain, sleep disruption, and cardiovascular risk. Cortisol is one of the four hormones identified in this book as the underlying chemistry of non-hunger eating.

C-REACTIVE PROTEIN (HIGH-SENSITIVITY, hsCRP)

A blood test that measures inflammation in the body at a level of sensitivity high enough to detect the chronic low-grade inflammation associated with metabolic disease. Optimal: below 1.0 mg/L. Elevated values indicate an inflammatory state that needs addressing.

DIABETES, TYPE 1

An autoimmune disease in which the immune system destroys the beta cells of the pancreas, leaving the patient unable to produce sufficient insulin. Distinct from type 2 diabetes. Requires lifelong insulin replacement. Not the disease this book is designed to reverse.

DIABETES, TYPE 2

A disease characterized by insulin resistance and progressive beta cell decline, resulting in elevated blood sugar. The disease this book is built to address. Reversible in many patients through the framework taught in these pages.

DIABETES REMISSION

A state defined in a consensus report as an A1C below 6.5 percent for at least three months without the use of glucose-lowering medications. The clinical destination of the work in this book for many patients.

FASTING GLUCOSE

The level of glucose in your blood after at least eight hours without food. Typically tested in the morning before breakfast. Normal: 70 to 99 mg/dL. Prediabetes: 100 to 125 mg/dL. Diabetes: 126 mg/dL and above.

FASTING INSULIN

The level of insulin in your blood after at least eight hours without food. An underutilized test that can reveal insulin resistance years before glucose values become abnormal. Optimal: below 10 μIU/mL.

FATTY LIVER (MASLD, formerly NAFLD)

A condition in which fat accumulates in the liver as a consequence of chronic insulin elevation and metabolic dysfunction. Strongly associated with type 2 diabetes. Often reversible with the same lifestyle interventions that reverse diabetes.

An international consensus of liver disease specialists formally renamed this condition. What was for decades called *non-alcoholic fatty liver disease* (NAFLD) is now called **MASLD** – *metabolic dysfunction-associated steatotic liver disease*. The new name is more accurate. The condition is not defined by the absence of alcohol. It is defined by the presence of metabolic dysfunction. The more severe inflammatory form, formerly known as NASH, is now called **MASH** – *metabolic dysfunction-associated steatohepatitis*. You may still see the older NAFLD and NASH terms in older literature and on some lab reports during the transition, but the current standard names are MASLD and MASH.

FOUR FORCES *

The four drivers of non-hunger eating identified by the H.E.A.T. model. See H.E.A.T.

GHRELIN

The hunger hormone. Released by the stomach when it is empty. Rises before meals and after periods of poor sleep. Causes a powerful drive to eat that is largely independent of conscious control. One of the four hormones identified in this book as the underlying chemistry of non-hunger eating.

GLP-1 (GLUCAGON-LIKE PEPTIDE 1)

A hormone released by the gut after a meal. Slows stomach emptying, increases satiety, and signals the pancreas to release insulin. The class of medications known as GLP-1 receptor agonists mimic and amplify this hormone's natural effects. Used for diabetes management and weight loss. Powerful tools, not substitutes for the framework taught here.

GLYCOGEN

The form in which the body stores glucose for short-term energy needs. Stored primarily in the liver and muscles. The body draws on glycogen stores between meals and during exercise.

H.E.A.T. *

A model identifying the four forces behind non-hunger eating: Habit (automatic behaviors triggered by environment), Emotion (eating to manage feelings rather than respond to hunger), Access (the proximity and ease of unhealthy food in your environment), and Taste (neurological reward responses to specific food categories). Each driver is addressed differently. The model is a diagnostic tool for understanding why you eat the way you eat.

HDL CHOLESTEROL

High-density lipoprotein cholesterol, often called "good" cholesterol because higher levels are associated with lower cardiovascular risk. Goal in metabolic health: above 60 mg/dL. Low HDL is one of the more reliable markers of insulin resistance.

HEPATIC

Relating to the liver.

HOMA-IR (HOMEOSTATIC MODEL ASSESSMENT OF INSULIN RESISTANCE)

A calculated value that estimates insulin resistance using fasting glucose and fasting insulin together. Below 1.5 is optimal. Above 2.0 indicates clinically significant resistance. A useful single number for tracking progress over time.

HORMONE

A chemical messenger produced by one part of the body and carried in the blood to affect another part. Insulin, cortisol, ghrelin, leptin, and the thyroid hormones are all examples. Hormones operate underneath the level of conscious thought and govern much of what we experience as appetite, mood, energy, and metabolism.

HYPERGLYCEMIA

Blood sugar that is higher than normal. The defining feature of untreated diabetes.

HYPERINSULINEMIA

Insulin levels that are higher than normal. Often present for years before blood sugar becomes elevated. One of the earliest signs that insulin resistance is developing.

HYPERPALATABLE

Engineered to be unusually rewarding to eat. A category of foods designed by the food industry to combine specific ratios of fat, sugar, salt, and texture that the brain's reward system finds difficult to resist. Most ultra-processed foods are hyperpalatable by design.

HYPOGLYCEMIA

Blood sugar that is lower than normal. Causes shakiness, sweating, confusion, and, in severe cases, loss of consciousness. A risk for patients on insulin or sulfonylurea medications, particularly as the framework in this book begins to reduce the body's need for these medications.

INSULIN

The hormone produced by the beta cells of the pancreas. Released in response to rising blood sugar. Signals the body's cells to absorb glucose from the blood, which lowers blood sugar levels. Also signals the body to store fat. The central hormone in the metabolic story this book tells.

INSULIN RESISTANCE

A state in which the body's cells become less responsive to insulin's signal. The pancreas compensates by producing more insulin. Over time, this compensation fails, blood sugar begins to rise, and type 2 diabetes develops. Insulin resistance is the root mechanism of metabolic disease and the primary target of the framework in this book.

LDL CHOLESTEROL

Low-density lipoprotein cholesterol. The cholesterol fraction most associated with cardiovascular disease, though the relationship is more nuanced than commonly presented. ApoB is generally a more accurate marker.

LEPTIN

The satiety hormone. Released by fat cells. Signals the brain that the body has enough stored energy and that eating can stop. Leptin resistance, in which the brain stops responding to leptin's signal, develops in many patients with insulin resistance and contributes to chronic overeating despite adequate fat stores.

METABOLIC SYNDROME

A cluster of conditions, including elevated blood sugar, abdominal obesity, high triglycerides, low HDL, and elevated blood pressure, that together significantly increase the risk of cardiovascular disease and type 2 diabetes. A patient meeting three or more of the criteria has metabolic syndrome.

METFORMIN

The most commonly prescribed first-line medication for type 2 diabetes. Reduces glucose production by the liver and improves insulin sensitivity. Generally well tolerated. Often discontinued during the reversal process as the body's underlying metabolism normalizes.

MICROALBUMIN

A protein that appears in the urine when the kidneys begin to leak. An early marker of diabetic kidney disease. Tested through a simple urine sample.

NON-HDL CHOLESTEROL

Total cholesterol minus HDL cholesterol. A more predictive marker of cardiovascular risk than LDL alone. Goal: below 130 mg/dL.

PANCREAS

The organ behind the stomach that produces insulin (in its beta cells) and several other hormones. Also produces digestive enzymes. The central organ in the metabolic story of diabetes.

POSTPRANDIAL

After a meal. A postprandial blood sugar reading is taken after eating, usually one or two hours after the meal began. Useful for understanding how specific foods affect your blood sugar.

POLYPHAGIA

Excessive hunger or increased appetite beyond what the body actually needs for energy. Polyphagia is one of the three classic recognized symptoms of diabetes, alongside excessive thirst and frequent urination. In type 2 diabetes, polyphagia arises not from caloric need but from a disease process in which cells cannot properly absorb glucose, causing the brain to continue generating hunger signals even when adequate calories have been consumed. Unlike conditioned hunger, which typically softens with time and responds to behavioral tools, polyphagia is driven by broken physiology and requires a different response. See Chapter Five.

PREDIABETES

A state in which blood sugar is elevated above normal but has not yet crossed the threshold for type 2 diabetes. Defined by an A1C between 5.7 and 6.4 percent, or a fasting glucose between 100 and 125 mg/dL. A warning state. Reversible with intervention.

REACTANCE

A well-documented psychological principle. The brain interprets a prohibition as a threat to its freedom and responds by leaning toward the forbidden thing. The reason diet protocols built on don't almost always fail in the long run. The framework in this book addresses food behavior by changing conditions rather than by issuing prohibitions.

SEVEN PILLARS *

The seven foundational practices of metabolic health taught in this book: walking, balanced bites, strength training, fasting, rest and recovery, mental mastery, and structure and planning. Together they form the daily infrastructure that sustains the framework over time.

SULFONYLUREA

A class of older diabetes medications that work by stimulating the pancreas to produce more insulin. Includes glipizide, glyburide, and glimepiride. Effective at lowering blood sugar but can cause hypoglycemia. Often reduced or discontinued during the reversal process.

TRIGLYCERIDE

A type of fat in the blood. Produced by the liver from excess carbohydrate. Elevated triglycerides are one of the more reliable signs of insulin resistance. Goal in metabolic health: below 100 mg/dL.

TRIGLYCERIDE-TO-HDL RATIO

A simple division: triglycerides divided by HDL. One of the better surrogate markers for insulin resistance available from a standard lipid panel. Below 2.0 is optimal. Above 3.0 strongly suggests insulin resistance.

TSH (THYROID STIMULATING HORMONE)

A pituitary hormone that signals the thyroid gland to produce thyroid hormone. The first-line test for thyroid dysfunction. Standard reference range: approximately 0.4 to 4.5 mIU/L.

URIC ACID

A byproduct of fructose metabolism and certain other dietary patterns. Elevated uric acid is associated with insulin resistance, fatty liver, hypertension, and gout. Often reduced significantly by reducing dietary fructose.

VISCERAL FAT

The fat stored deep in the abdomen, surrounding internal organs. Distinct from subcutaneous fat (the fat beneath the skin). Visceral fat is metabolically active and is strongly associated with insulin resistance and cardiovascular risk.

VITAMIN D (25-HYDROXYVITAMIN D)

The stored form of vitamin D, used as the standard measure of vitamin D status. Optimal range: 50 to 80 ng/mL. Deficiency is associated with insulin resistance and a wide range of other conditions.

WOODE LIFE DESIGN *

The educational and personal development platform on which the framework in this book is taught and practiced. Includes the Weekly Brief email newsletter, the Accelerators community, video content, and the broader publishing and clinical work that supports it.

NOTES

Notes are keyed to chapter and page. For the reader's convenience, the most important sources are listed first.

CHAPTER ONE

1. ADA 2021 consensus on diabetes remission criteria: Riddle MC, Cefalu WT, Evans PH, et al. "Consensus Report: Definition and Interpretation of Remission in Type 2 Diabetes." *Diabetes Care*. October 2021;44(10):2438--2444. https://doi.org/10.2337/dci21-0034. Representing the American Diabetes Association, the Endocrine Society, the European Association for the Study of Diabetes, and Diabetes UK. Published simultaneously in *The Journal of Clinical Endocrinology & Metabolism*, *Diabetologia*, and *Diabetic Medicine*. Note: This is a consensus report representing expert opinion; it is not an ADA position statement or treatment guideline. A prior ADA consensus statement (2009) introduced the term "remission"; the 2021 report established more rigorous and widely endorsed criteria.

2. DiRECT trial — primary clinical evidence for lifestyle-induced remission: Lean ME, Leslie WS, Barnes AC, et al. "Primary care-led weight management for remission of type 2 diabetes (DiRECT): an open-label, cluster-randomised trial." *Lancet*. 2018;391(10120):541--551. https://doi.org/10.1016/S0140-6736(17)33102-1. At 12 months, 46% of the intervention group achieved remission; 36% remained in remission at 24 months (Lean MEJ et al. *Lancet Diabetes Endocrinol*. 2019;7(5):344--355). Five-year extension data published 2024 (Lean MEJ et al. *Lancet Diabetes Endocrinol*). Note: DiRECT used an intensive low-calorie diet (825--853 kcal/day) in participants with diabetes duration under six years; remission durability is linked to sustained weight loss.

CHAPTER THREE

3. The "bliss point" and Howard Moskowitz's research: Moss M. *Salt Sugar Fat: How the Food Giants Hooked Us*. New York: Random House; 2013.

CHAPTER FOUR

4. Exercise-induced glucose uptake via GLUT4 independent of insulin: Richter EA, Hargreaves M. "Exercise, GLUT4, and Skeletal Muscle Glucose Uptake." *Physiological Reviews*. 2013;93(3):993--1017.

CHAPTER FIVE

5. Sleep deprivation and appetite hormones: Spiegel K, Tasali E, Penev P, Van Cauter E. *Annals of Internal Medicine*. 2004;141(11):846--850.

6. GLP-1 receptor agonists: see the current *ADA Standards of Medical Care in Diabetes*, updated annually at diabetes.org.

CHAPTER TEN

7. Kitchen environment and food behavior (Chapter Ten): The body of research supporting environmental food cues is robust and well-established across multiple independent investigators.

8. Postprandial satiety and polyphagia in type 2 diabetes (Chapter Five): Knudsen SH, Hansen LS, Pedersen M, et al. "Effects of 2 weeks of interval training on glucose handling in participants with type 2 diabetes." Journal of Applied Physiology. 2013;116(12):1484–1492. For hyperglycemia and postprandial satiety hormone suppression, see: Moulin CM, Rizzo LV, Calliari LE, et al. "Glucagon-like peptide-1 and peptide YY responses to a meal are attenuated in obese subjects with type 2 diabetes." American Journal of Physiology-Endocrinology and Metabolism. 2014;308(6):E489–E496. These sources support the clinical description of hunger worsening or failing to resolve postprandially in patients with type 2 diabetes, including the Layer 4 satiety signal failure described in Chapter Five.

9. Hypothalamic hunger signaling and prefrontal cortex structure (Chapter Five): For the structural relationship between hypothalamic hunger circuits and prefrontal cortical function, see: Lowe CJ, Morton JB, Reichelt AC. "Adolescent obesity and dietary decision making—a brain health perspective." The Lancet Child and Adolescent Health. 2020;4(5):388–396; and Carnell S, Gibson C, Benson L, et al. "Neuroimaging and obesity: current knowledge and future directions." Obesity Reviews. 2012;13(1):43–56. The relationship between hypothalamic hunger signaling and prefrontal cortical function reflects converging findings across metabolic neuroscience, including structural and functional associations observed in neuroimaging studies of obesity and appetite dysregulation.

10. Protein intake and endogenous GLP-1 release (Chapter Five): Protein-rich foods stimulate GLP-1 secretion through calcium-sensing receptors and amino acid sensing in intestinal L-cells. See: Lejeune MP, Westerterp KR, Adam TC, et al. "Ghrelin and glucagon-like peptide 1 concentrations, 24-h satiety, and energy and substrate metabolism during a high-protein diet and measured in a respiration chamber." American Journal of Clinical Nutrition. 2006;83(1):89–94.

CHAPTER SIX

11. Whole fruit versus fruit juice and type 2 diabetes risk: Muraki I, Imamura F, Manson JE, et al. "Fruit consumption and risk of type 2 diabetes: results from three prospective longitudinal cohort studies." *BMJ.* 2013;347:f5001. https://doi.org/10.1136/bmj.f5001. Greater whole-fruit intake — particularly blueberries, grapes, and apples — was associated with lower risk, while greater fruit-juice intake was associated with higher risk, consistent with the role of intact fiber and food structure in moderating the glycemic impact of naturally occurring sugars. The added-sugar amounts cited in this chapter (in seasonings, sauces, granolas, and bars) are drawn from product nutrition labels and vary by brand.

CHAPTER EIGHT

12. Cortisol and the drive toward high-calorie "comfort" food: Dallman MF, Pecoraro N, Akana SF, et al. "Chronic stress and obesity: a new view of 'comfort food.'" *Proceedings of the National Academy of Sciences.* 2003;100(20):11696–11701. https://doi.org/10.1073/pnas.1934666100.

13. The hypothalamic-pituitary-adrenal (HPA) axis and the physiology of chronic stress: Chrousos GP. "Stress and disorders of the stress system." *Nature Reviews Endocrinology.* 2009;5(7):374–381. https://doi.org/10.1038/nrendo.2009.106.

CHAPTER NINE

14. The "amygdala hijack": the term was coined by Daniel Goleman, drawing on the work of Joseph LeDoux. Goleman D. *Emotional Intelligence: Why It Can Matter More Than IQ.* New York: Bantam Books; 1995.

15. Affect labeling — putting feelings into words — and reduced amygdala activity (the basis for the Clarify step): Lieberman MD, Eisenberger NI, Crockett MJ, et al.

"Putting Feelings Into Words: Affect Labeling Disrupts Amygdala Activity in Response to Affective Stimuli." *Psychological Science.* 2007;18(5):421–428. https://doi.org/10.1111/j.1467-9280.2007.01916.x.

16. The two-system model of fast, automatic thinking and slow, deliberate thinking that underlies the Pause: Kahneman D. *Thinking, Fast and Slow.* New York: Farrar, Straus and Giroux; 2011.

A NOTE ON CITATIONS

This book is written for patients, not clinicians. Citations are provided for key foundational claims and for any statistic or study attributed to a specific source. General mechanistic descriptions reflect well-established endocrinological principles and standard clinical teaching. Readers seeking the primary research literature are directed to the ADA's Standards of Medical Care in Diabetes and the references therein.

www.ingramcontent.com/pod-product-compliance
Lightning Source LLC
LaVergne TN
LVHW091158150826
845672LV00005B/1189

* 9 7 9 8 9 9 5 9 1 5 6 0 7 *